WHAT THEY ARE SAYING About *Essential Environments* . . .

"Essential Environments is exactly what I have been looking for to provide our clients with a beautiful source book for healing their homes and living spaces. This book paves the way for the current renaissance in healthy, simple living."

—LAWRENCE AXIL COMRAS
Founder & President
Greenhome.com

"A lifestyle that is tuned into one's natural environment can bring joy to everyday activities. The products that we buy, eat and drive matter. Janie Quinn reminds us of this without being judgmental or dogmatic—she shows us how to be good and have fun too!"

—BONNIE BARKETT, SENIOR POLICY ADVISOR
United States Environmental Protection Agency

"If you want guidance on how to live without harming yourself and the planet, this book provides it. Quinn gets right down to business, offering concrete suggestions for what one can do to ensure a healthy lifestyle while at the same time contributing to the ecological health of our planet."

—CHRIS UHL, PH.D.
Professor , Penn State University
and author of Developing Ecological Consciousness

"A must read if you're trying to rid your life of toxicity and cure daily diseases. As Recreation Chairman of the Susquehanna River Watch, I can see that the suggestions in this book will make a difference in cleaning up the waterways of our country and the waterways of your life."

—GERALD M. REISINGER, N.D.
Specializing in Preventative Medicine
Kingston, Pennsylvania

"Essential Environments makes the complicated, scientific realm of environmental protection within your reach by suggesting steps that each of us can take for the collective good. Consider it."

—JO-ELLEN DARCY, SENIOR POLICY ADVISOR
Committee on Environment and Public Works,
United States Senate

"Essential Environments is a comprehensive guide that provides the necessary knowledge to both understand the risks within the environments people live in and make choices to create change that benefits all. I highly recommend it."

—JEFFREY HOLLENDER
CEO Seventh Generation
and author of What Matters Most

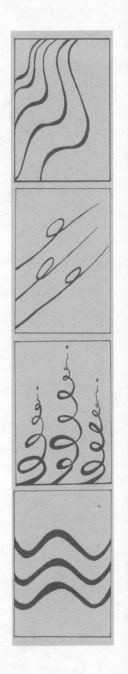

Essential Environments

Essential Environments™

Discover How to Create
Healthy Living Spaces

Janie Quinn
Environmental Consultant and
Award-winning Author of Essential Eating

AZURE MOON PUBLISHING
Waverly, Pennsylvania
www.essentialliving.com

Published by Azure Moon Publishing
Post Office Box 771, Waverly, PA 18471

For information or additional books:
(570) 586-1557
essentialliving.com

Editors: Lee Ann Cavanaugh & Pattie Franks-Evanish
Book Design: North Market Street Graphics
Photography: Kathryn LeSoine
Illustrator: Valerie Kiser

Publisher's Cataloging-in Publication Data
Quinn, Janie.
Essential environments : discover how to create
healthy living spaces / Janie Quinn.—1st ed.
p.   cm.
Includes bibliographical references and index.
LCCN 2004107281
ISBN 0-9679843-8-6
1. Housing and health.   2. Indoor air pollution—
Prevention.   3. Household supplies—Toxicology.
4. Consumer product safety.   I. Title.
RA770.5.Q56   2004   640
QBI33-2054

Printed in the United States of America on 100% post-consumer recycled, EcoBook paper using vegetable based ink.

To the earth, the air, the water, and the wildlife,
to the past, present and future,
to our global relatives,
and most importantly, to you!
May your world become a healthier space.

PROLOGUE—THE ALPHA MONKEY

The synchronicity of life has always amazed me. Upon completing this book I realized that this year, 2004, is the Chinese Year of The Monkey. There is no coincidence that I had already included two stories about monkeys—one in this prologue and the other in the epilogue. As the closest species to humans, monkeys are often studied and observed so we can learn from their behavior.

Years ago, a group of scientists was observing the behavior patterns of a colony of monkeys deep in the jungle. Early on, they began to notice that a particular monkey appeared to be sitting apart from the group. In a few weeks, they had recorded enough consistent evidence to confirm that each day this monkey spent time separated from the colony. It would often sit gazing upon the horizon.

The scientists conferred and agreed that this monkey was definitely showing classical signs of depression. The researchers decided to intercede in order to help the monkey develop into an active member of the group. Within a few days, the monkey was captured and taken back to civilization to be rehabilitated and encouraged out of his suspected depression.

Six months later, the scientists determined that, although no progress or improvement was visible, it was time to return the monkey to his colony in the jungle. Upon arriving in the region where they captured the monkey, they were shocked at what they found. All the monkeys in the colony were dead.

Gradually, the scientists then began to comprehend what had occurred, although it was much too late. They recognized the poignant fact that the monkey

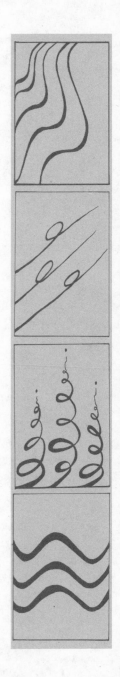

they had removed from the colony was the "alpha" monkey. In animal packs or colonies, the alpha animals are responsible for protecting the group by warning them of danger—warning them when a predator is near, warning them when a threatening storm is approaching. By removing the alpha monkey, the colony was left exposed and unprotected.

Essential Environments is your alpha guide for a sustainable, healthy life. Similar to the alpha animal, it will help you to recognize and reduce the impending dangers and harmful toxins in your world. The delicate balance of nature's rhythm emerges from essential environments and teaches us to believe in ourselves and each other. You can save yourself. We can save each other.

CONTENTS

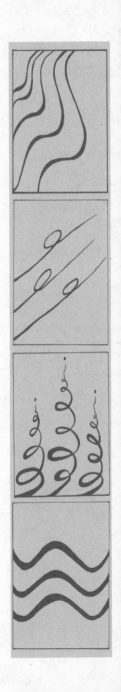

Chapter 2 ⚊ EARTH   15

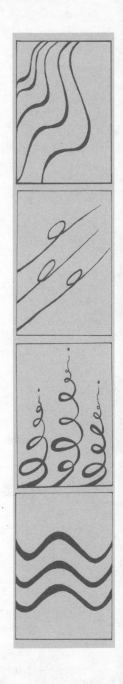

AUTHOR'S NOTE

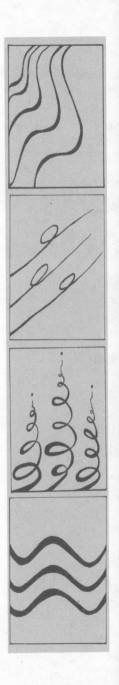

Not all dreams are made to be chased—some are intended to be captured. I have an incredible dream of a healthful, life-sustaining world where humans, animals and plants thrive in harmony with the flow of nature. The beauty of dreaming is that the impossible is possible. History provides us with a wealth of incredible dreamers whose dreams came true. Saint Francis of Assisi, known for his deep respect and kindness to animals and nature, inspires us with his words—start by doing what's necessary, then what's possible and suddenly you are doing the impossible. When pursuing one's dream with intention and perseverance, anything is possible. *Essential Environments,* a dream that is possible, is a guide for protecting and sustaining yourself and your world, because you matter and your environment matters.

The gift of *Essential Environments* continues to show me the divine in simple things. I feel that I have been chosen to be the messenger for these simple truths that I myself needed to learn. These simple truths helped heal my life and awakened me to the fact that unless I saved myself first, I surely did not have a chance of rescuing my children and those that I love or safeguarding our earth. Now, I happily share this gift with you.

A deluge of books have been written about our environment, however, few offer simple steps that encourage an individual to consider change in such a positive way. This book was conceived after years of creating essential environments and studying how to safeguard our health from the insidious onslaught of chemicals in our lives. I do not pretend to be an expert in all fields, although my experience, research and trial and error have helped me to become an expert in living a healthy life through eating real foods and avoiding unnecessary chemicals.

I am constantly inspired to be a more conscious consumer and global citizen; however, I could be better. There are things in this book that I have yet to incorporate into my life, but I am aspiring to that goal. This information will help you to begin saving yourself from the daily assault of chemicals and to promote sustainable life here on earth. The solutions to complicated problems often start with a single step—*all* of our single steps.

Please join me in taking the next simple step toward cleaning "your home," dreaming the impossible dream and healing yourself. Enjoy the journey. It can be an exciting one.

Essential Environments

Chapter 1

You & Your Space

You & Your Space

Essential Environments is your guidebook for creating healthy living spaces that nurture your health, your family's health and the health of your pets. It is for everyone, especially those who are beginning to realize the need to guard and protect themselves and their world from the daily chemical assault and the exhaustion of our resources. This information will help you create a positive difference in your world and awaken to the vast benefits of becoming a more conscientious inhabitant of our Earth.

Essential Environments simplifies the complexity of our environmental issues by dividing them into single servings, one day at a time, and one page at a time and, most importantly, one consideration at a time. If you find yourself becoming overwhelmed by the scope of this book, I suggest you use it as you would a cookbook. Flip through the pages until you find a morsel of information that resonates with your "tastes." Then consider incorporating this solution into your lifestyle. When you feel comfortable with your initial consideration and are ready for another step, read and absorb another page. Proceed at your own pace; a small step today will make your life easier tomorrow. All of our little changes will eventually add up to be big ones.

A small step today will make your life easier tomorrow.

According to the U.S. Census Bureau, the average American moves 11.7 times in a lifetime. More than ever before in our history as a people, our Society is disconnected from the earth and the flow of nature and it is causing disorder in our lives. We spend almost 95 percent of our time in man-made environments further disconnecting us from the balance of nature. Nearly all of our living structures are created and maintained with chemical-laden substances that do not support human health or balance nature's effects.

We instinctively know that nature provides a positive healing force in our lives. Consider the fact that we send our troubled youth to "wilderness" camps in order to heal their character defects. If the call of the outdoors is not real, then why do we sit inside longingly looking out the window, watching the snow fall or daydreaming about a summer afternoon picnic? *Essential Environments* emphasizes that nature is a priceless human resource that is worthy of being honored. There is much to be learned from the natural world and the indigenous societies that honored and understood the value of our natural resources and personal health.

On your daily path of life, you register an average of 36,000 images, both consciously and subconsciously; and you have an estimated 65,000 thoughts. From the moment you wake up in the morning until you return home, the symbols, artifacts, colors, air quality and things in your path create your intentions, your focus and your dreams. What does your path look like? What images are you looking at every day? Who is on your path with you? What activities do you promote on your path? Where is your path taking you? For example, if your closets are stuffed, your life may be blocked. If you pull into your garage and are welcomed by cans of toxic chemicals, your life may be toxic. If the air in your bedroom is stagnant, something in your life may be stagnant. If your pantry is filled with junk food, your health is not a high priority. The considerations and motivations in *Essential Environments* are offered as a guide to inspire us all to remove the clutter from our lives, to use fewer resources, to avoid toxic chemicals and to promote sustainable practices. Incorporating these earth- and human-friendly actions into your path of life will help you to create a cleaner, more nourishing, sustainable path.

Complex political, social and cultural views often cloud the environmental discussion. There are many publications that bring these problems to light. *Essential Environments* touches on these issues but focuses instead on individual solutions that can easily be incorporated into your daily life. All of our small steps will collectively impact the global problems like over population, militarization, media violence, over consumption, global warming, natural resource depletion and other issues that tend to overwhelm an individual. Take very small steps if you need to; just be certain you take them. Weigh the benefits and disadvantages of harmful chemicals and decide for yourself. Most often there isn't a perfect solution, just a better choice. Connecting to and purifying your personal environments will initiate and support the changes desired in our global community.

Considering Change

Considering is an essential word when contemplating change. The first step in healing and becoming healthy is not change. The first step is *considering* that change could take place—considering that you could live on a healthy planet and in a healthy body. *Considering*, not changing, is your starting point. The suggestion of *considering* can break down the barrier of fear that inhibits change. Although faced with it daily, change is what humans fear the most. Start by *considering* as it does not require or demand change.

As you read these suggestions for toxic-free living just *consider* that you could participate. Reversing the tide toward living without toxicity may seem overwhelming, but consider starting with a simple baby step such as buying chemical-free toothpaste. Consider how just one tiny step will be easier than the daily ritual of living with dis-ease.

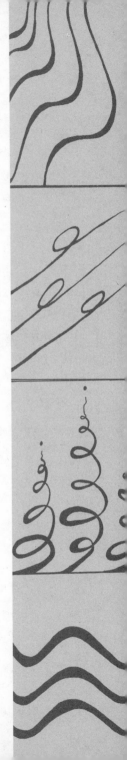

You can declare a gradual defense against the perils of a world gone progressively toxic; or you can choose to remain a victim to the environmental assaults that enter and negatively affect our lives. Either way, *you are* making a choice!

Environmental issues can sometimes evoke feelings of resistance. This resistance is not directed toward the idea of toxic-free living but toward the actual life adjustment it would require. In this case, the fringe benefits of these changes will certainly alter your life in a positive, healthy, and humanistic manner. *Essential Environments* focuses on what could be done and what should be done. It is in not a textbook, but an instructional guide with considerations for upgrading your quality of life, health, and environment.

Poor health brought me face-to-face with the need to change. First, I considered that I could remove at least some of the harmful chemicals and toxicity from my life. Then, baby step by baby step, I became a better consumer by purchasing toxic-free products from environmentally-friendly companies. I found that many of these products were available through local businesses.

Overwhelmed by the idea of changing *the* world, I just changed *my* world. We, as humans, have always possessed the power to create and to destroy; but more importantly, we also possess the power to sustain and to rebuild both our lives and of those around us. Gradually, through baby steps, my home and office became clean and green spaces. The *environment* healed and I healed. Those around me saw the transformation and considered that they too could experience the benefits of clean and green spaces. Then they *considered* changing. They *changed*. They *healed*.

Overwhelmed by the idea of changing the world, I just changed my world.

Your Daily Diseases

Most people do not associate the dis-ease in their body with the chemicals that have been added to our planet in the last fifty-odd years. According to Environmental Protection Agency's Toxic Substance Control Act inventory, there are presently 80,000 harmful chemicals in existence. Think about the increase in serious illnesses such as obesity, cancer, cardiovascular disease, thyroid disease, autoimmune diseases, diabetes, infertility, allergies, asthma, migraines, attention deficit hyperactivity disorder, arthritis, celiac disease, depression, indigestion and more. The escalation of dis-ease is a reaction to the chemicals that have been added to our food, water and air supply, thereby weakening the body's defenses.

Your daily dis-ease can be greatly reduced by eliminating the sources of toxins from of your life. It is much easier than you think and you are worth it. Consider living in a state of ease, not dis-ease. *Essential Environments* shows you how to reclaim your right to healthy food, air and water, one page at a time.

As with all things, achieving a balance is essential. Advocating the elimination of chemicals from our daily lives is not what this book is expressing or communicating. Chemicals have certainly made numerous impressive and fantastic advances in our culture and time. The major concern being highlighted here is that chemicals are used too frequently as the first approach to a problem. Through irresponsible overuse and overextension, chemicals have invaded and unbalanced both our ecosystem and our bodies. *Essential Environments* helps you to decide the level of toxicity and daily dis-ease you are willing to accept.

Simplifying Your Choices

Over the last decade, I have continued to seek out and embrace ways to simplify my life. This does not translate into just organizing my life, but identifying, simplifying, and managing the multitude of endless choices that confront us day after day. Think about the time and effort it takes to choose between 360 hair-care products or 40 varieties of toothpaste on your grocery store shelf. As our choices increase, uncertainties escalate making it easy to become overloaded and confused to the point of being paralyzed.

In our express lane culture, the time to contemplate or reflect upon our choices is extremely limited. This inevitably leads to excess—excess stuff, excess people, and excess commitments that just complicate our lives. Wanting very badly to stop the excesses and the excuses, I pledged to live my life guided by what I call Absolute Choices. Now when I am confronted with multiple options, my decision is frequently made as a result of simplification. By simplifying my basic choices, I experienced less indecision and anxiety and discovered leisure time to enjoy my healthier and happier lifestyle.

The first Absolute Choice to simplify life is to eat real food—that is, food which is free of chemicals and is not processed. After all, every experience is improved and every performance or accomplishment feels enhanced when we live in a healthy body. When I began to eat real food, something quite incredible occurred; my health was restored! I lost excess weight and found myself bursting with an abundance of energy. Knowing what

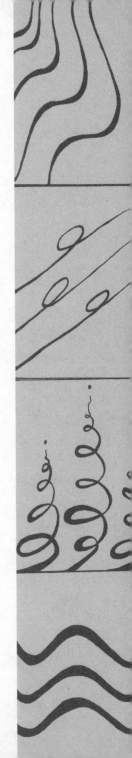

is safe and nourishing to eat is the simple principle that allows us the freedom of having a healthy body.

I soon began to realize it was not only the fake food that was creating the disorder and dis-ease in my life. My research finally led me to acknowledge the undeniable connection between the 80,000 chemicals that have been added to our ecosystem and the epidemic of serious illness in America.

Therefore, the second Absolute Choice for simplifying life is to diminish your exposure to harmful chemicals in order to create safe, healthy, and healing environments in which to inhabit. Reducing the variety of products needed to clean and maintain my living and working spaces has helped simplify my life. Buying less things and replacing products with earth- and human-friendly products also reduces shopping time and saves money. My choice to reduce these chemicals has had a far reaching effect in all areas of my life from eliminating my need for allergy medicine to enjoying a thriving garden. By gradually establishing two Absolute Choices—to eat real food and reduce the harmful chemicals in my life, I easily found more free time and created a healthy refuge in which to live.

I may not know you, but I am very proud of you. I am proud that you are considering saving yourself by eating foods and creating environments that support your health. Although it is not always easy, it is always worth it. Best-selling author Matthew Kelly writes that your choices create your habits, your habits create your character and your character creates your destiny. I applaud you for considering that you can make better choices to save your destiny from pollution and dis-ease.

The art of self-love is not about conceit, but about knowing yourself.

Love & Save Yourself

Loving yourself is the foundation for creating your essential environment and fueling your body for peak performance. We have truly forgotten how to love ourselves. Our culture supports taking care of the needs of others before our own. The truth is that unless you love yourself first, you cannot really fully love others. The art of self-love is not about conceit, but about knowing yourself. Knowing your needs, your desires, and your dreams creates a better you. Loving yourself is not selfish, it is smart.

Often I am asked the question, "How do you do all this with a family, and a busy career?" The answer is easy—you save yourself first. By placing yourself first and saving yourself first, you will become a wonderful example to your family and friends. Practicing this self-love philosophy, not promoting it, is the key. I found that by creating safe, healthy spaces and fueling my body with real food created a beacon signaling others to do the same.

Airlines are great examples of the save yourself first principle. In case of an emergency, airlines instruct adults to put on their oxygen mask first, before helping others. They know that if you get oxygen to support your own brain function first then you, and others have a better chance of survival. You can not save anyone else if you do not save yourself first. You are worth it and so are they!

Environmental Disorder—Chemical Sensitivity

Fifteen percent of our population today suffers from sensitivity to environmental chemicals, a malady known as Multiple Chemical Sensitivity (MCS) disorder. Because MCS sufferers experience a multitude of symptoms, diagnosis can be difficult. MCS is now recognized as a disability and symptoms range from not being able to leave the house to being allergic to perfume. Since MCS is triggered by exposure to chemicals, it is not surprising that there is a noticeable increase in this disorder, considering most of the chemicals used in consumer products have not been tested for health effects or the impact of low-level, long-term exposure.

The MSC disorder is spawning new governmental regulations for air and water quality control in the workplace, but change is agonizingly slow. Unfortunately ignorance and greed often prevent companies from realizing that the benefits of essential environments are intricately and eternally interconnected to the success of their business. The real change is coming from companies that recognize the worthwhile investment of creating safe, healthy environments in the workplace for their employees.

It was no coincidence that during my journey of writing this book, my friend, Jean, was placed in my path to share in my search of how to create healthy environments. Ten years ago Jean was stricken with MCS. Doctors were unable to diagnose her symptoms. She became seriously ill and almost died. By using the considerations in this book to remove the harmful chemicals from her life and combining reflexology treatments each day saved her life. Today, Jean lives an essential life as a certified reflexologist who is widening the path for others that are considering a chemical-free life.

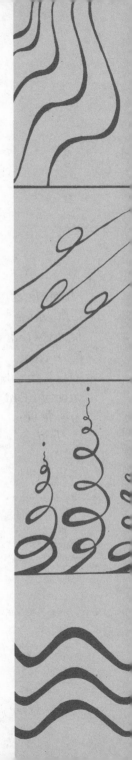

Essential Eating

Prior to the widespread use of chemicals in agriculture and modern food processing, we innately knew how to eat real, nutritious food that supported our health and enhanced our lives without damaging our habitats. Today, finding and choosing natural versus chemical-laden foods can be an adventure, a worthwhile adventure. Chapter Four addresses how to get the chemicals out of your eating lifestyle and how to put real food back into your diet.

As a prelude to *Essential Environments*, I wrote *Essential Eating: Discover How To Eat, Not Diet*. It outlines an eating lifestyle that can create an essential environment inside your body. The transition from essential eating to essential environments was a natural progression because it is impossible to live in a healthy body and not be aware of and affected by the surrounding environment—the two are linked and cannot be treated as separate entities.

It outlines an eating lifestyle that can create an essential environment inside your body.

It is no mere coincidence that our young people are physically developing earlier than their predecessors due to the fact that growth hormones and other chemicals have been introduced as cornerstones in our food and water supply. More and more school-aged children are overweight, they wear synthetic clothing made from and laundered by chemicals, and occupy a room that has been cleaned with harmful chemicals. The real icing on the cake is that they drink chemically-treated sugar water, and eat processed food snacks throughout the day.

How can school children be expected to learn and function in this environment or should I say in spite of this environment? Grievously, this scenario is all too common for millions of children. The rise in Attention Deficit Disorder (ADD), Attention Deficit and Hyperactivity Disorder (ADHD), allergies, asthma, teenage migraines, headaches, stomach aches, ear infections, eating disorders, childhood diabetes, obesity, early onset of puberty and menstruation and a host of other diet- and environmentally-related sicknesses are not the side-effects, but the effects of the harmful chemicals in our world. *Essential Environments* offers solutions for changing this sad scenario for our children.

Truth in Knowing

It is not what you know; it is what you do not know that will kill you. The ideas presented in *Essential Environments* are not new; they are just not presently acknowledged and understood on a large enough scale. When these ideas begin to mainstream, we will have a healthier world, physically, mentally, emotionally and spiritually. For example, once you know that fragrances can cause headaches, allergies and/or neurological damage, use this knowledge to consider getting them out of your life.

Sometimes you just intuitively distinguish that something is true without proof. That is what I call *knowing*; like knowing that throwing litter out of a car window is wrong. You do not have proof, but you *know* it is wrong. Many of the ideas about saving the earth are instinctive—you just *know*. Knowing is taking the responsibility to respond and interact with your world on an instinctive human level.

Although much of the information in this book has been researched and proven, the overwhelming scientific data and terminology that can keep us from recognizing a simple solution has been kept to a minimum. I opted to provide you with simple solutions that resonate with *knowing* which goes beyond common sense. Everyone knows how to take care of Mother Earth on some level; therefore we need to awaken our senses to that intuition—that knowing. You are capable of knowing what is good for you.

Feng Shui, Ancient Art of Balance

A tree is never too fat, a river too long or a mountain too high. Nature provides us with an example of balance that creates harmony. If you have ever had the pleasure of being in the natural world without any man-made intrusions, then you have experienced the healing power of nature—the uninterrupted flow of being. Understanding nature's healing power and using it in your own environment is the art of Feng Shui.

This ancient art of bringing the balance of nature into our man-made environments is based on oldest book known to man—the *I Ching* or the *Book of Changes*. It explains that a balanced life is one that is lived with intention and with the flow of nature. It is easier than you might think. Your life probably already dictates partial participation in the flow of nature, such as dressing for the weather, eating foods that are in season and participating in seasonal activities. The key to living in the flow of nature is authenticity—undisputed credibility, truth, correctness, and being *genuine*.

In a society brimming with fake, inauthentic practices and products, being authentic can put more soulful meaning into life. For example, in nature pine trees do not have maple leaves and rocks do not have wings. A balanced, natural world does not encompass plastic materials, synthetic chemicals or artificial colors. Participating in sustainable

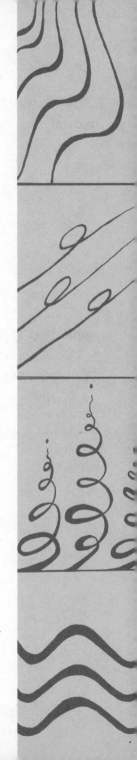

practices, eating real foods and reducing and eliminating the use of toxic products forms the foundation for your intention to be authentic and live with the flow of nature.

Many years ago a friend gave me a book about Feng Shui. Unaware that this 10,000 year old art even existed, I was amazed to discover that during my entire life I had possessed the *knowing* of Feng Shui principles. My thirst for Feng Shui knowledge led me to become a certified Feng Shui Consultant and to establish a company dedicated to creating healthy spaces and bringing harmony into man-made environments. We all understand Feng Shui on a certain level. It explains why we either feel comfortable or want to flee from a space.

Essential Environments is outlined according to four basic elements: earth, air, fire and water. When these elements are balanced in nature, harmony is created. The kind of harmonious energy that inspires you, recreates you, supports you and protects you. Feng Shui principles draw from these elements to organize and de-toxify spaces.

Use the healing properties of nature to create harmony in your man-made environments.

The Earth Chapter includes products and practices connected with household and industrial cleaning, bath and beauty treatments, flooring, lighting, automotive, lawn and garden, and other effects associated with your homes and your land. The Air Chapter is comprised of products and practices related to the air quality of an environment, air filtering and purification. The Water Chapter outlines products and practices that affect your water including filtration systems, water testing and how to protect your water quality. Finally, the Fire Chapter is associated with the fuel your body consumes. It discusses products and practices that will assist you in making better food and drug choices in order to support your health such as non-toxic foods, safe cookware, and solutions for diet-related diseases, healthy drinks and alternatives to prescription drugs. These four symbolic elements—earth, air, fire and water—remind you to use the healing properties of nature to create harmony in your man-made environments so they can accordingly support your health.

Industry Considers Change

Industries that are resistant to finding solutions to chemical manufacturing and chemical processing are in for a big surprise. Consumers are awakening and their purchasing power is directed toward clean and green products, companies and philosophies.

Consumers are becoming more conscious of the toxicity of foods grown by using traditional farming methods and, as a result, are buying more organic foods. In fact, due to increasing consumer demand, organic foods have become the largest growing segment in grocery stores. The key factor is that grocery stores did not decide to offer more organic food—it was generated by consumer demand. Without a doubt, the ripple effect of this is enormous. Farmers are now growing more organic products; therefore, fewer chemicals are being leached into the earth. Food manufacturers are diversifying their product lines to include and cater to organic foods and its advocates. Some companies are even embracing an organic mindset that celebrates their support of toxic-free living.

As an end result, food manufacturers are being challenged to provide real food that is free of chemicals, additives, colorings and flavorings. Many consumers have come to the realization that fast food is directly involved in the proliferation of obesity and are taking steps to make better choices. Consider that in your lifetime nutritionally deficient fast food could become extinct.

Another example of consumer-driven demand is the cooperative health care movement. Health care practitioners are learning about and including cooperative medicine and modalities in their practices because their patients are requesting it. Cooperative healing modalities such as reflexology, acupuncture and healing touch are becoming more mainstreamed due to consumer interest and satisfaction. Patients, not institutions or corporations, are motivating traditional medical practitioners to recognize and to secure training in the field of cooperative-healing modalities. Ask and you shall receive is the mantra for the transformations being initiated by the educated and enlightened consumer.

The motivations for our industries to develop embrace and adhere to a mandatory consciousness towards protecting and improving the environment are being consumer generated. You, as a consumer, have the right to insist that industries provide safe and natural environments that support your health and accomplish it through practices that support healing the earth. Our voices and our choices will eventually compel companies, manufacturers, and industries to be held accountable for their actions. Your purchases are counted as your vote. Consumers are awakening and claiming the power to restore their right to a clean and green world.

Raising Corporate & Consumer Consciousness

Environmental solutions that seem obvious and straightforward become thorny because of the costs involved. In order to do the right thing and correct these pressing problems, corporations need to be financially and morally accountable for the toxic trespasses of

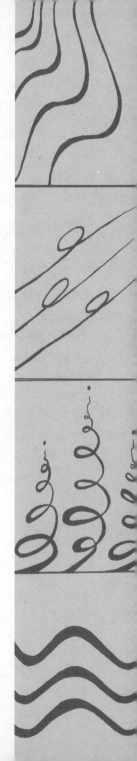

the past, as well as being responsible for any potentially detrimental future actions. Such corrective measures would cut into profit margins causing resistance and hesitation on the corporation's part. The worn-out excuse that the solutions to cleaning up our environment are cost-prohibitive and insurmountable is no longer acceptable. For a sustainable future we need to cultivate a conscience back into corporate decision-making.

You can make a difference by making healthier purchases. Start by purchasing goods that are clean, green, free and clear—goods that support life and protect you. This seemingly small personal preference increases the demand for more corporate environmental awareness. Consumer action can be much more devastating than any fines that are assessed upon companies for violating environmental codes and human ethics. Buying products close to home whenever possible indirectly benefits the environment while it subsequently reduces the amount of fuel used to transport them.

When questioned about the chemicals or procedures used in creating their products, we found most companies fell into two categories: companies that had a strong resistance to sharing this information and those that did not. It is no coincidence that the companies that easily shared their ingredients and practices were usually environmentally- and user-friendly. These companies were very proud of the fact that they are contributing to the solution of toxic-free living. The companies that refused to provide ingredients and discuss procedures were typically toxic. The companies that shared their information and produce earth- and user-friendly products are listed under the Sources Chapter.

Don't let fear paralyze you— let it be a catalyst for progressing, not retreating!

Be the Solution

Volumes have been written about the problem of toxins in our environment. It seems that the more I research the more bad news seems to surface. We have far too much excess information today—too much *fear based* information. The nature of fear is to provide you with just enough information to become fearful, but not enough information to dispel the fear or see beyond the crisis. Fear itself is a tendril that can bring into your life the very thing that you fear. Feelings of fear are restrictive and can keep you stuck in a fearful state. Don't let fear paralyze you—let it be a catalyst for progressing, not retreating!

Consider that excitement can be created when we face our fears. The type of excitement created as a result of becoming open and accepting to the changes in our lives such as new attitudes, new policies and new solutions for daily living. When choosing to consider these exciting changes, we are also choosing to consider the exciting solutions—solutions that can, if done collectively save the earth and ourselves.

One of the biggest challenges of *Essential Environments* is to present you with solutions for creating cleaner homes and working spaces without overwhelming you into paralysis and apathy. Since researching this book I have realized that it is virtually impossible for the human mind, including mine, to totally and completely comprehend the effects of pollution on our environment. Nearly all ecology books and articles focus on future projections that magnify the current situations into science-fiction like settings. I refuse to invite, tolerate or accept this mindset of hopelessness. Instead I believe that the solution lies in our collective awakening through making better choices and considering that a cleaner, healthier world is possible.

Essential Environments is structured to focus on solutions intended to rid the harmful chemicals from your life. In each of the respective chapters, Earth, Air, Fire and Water, each topic begins with a brief overview of the challenges related to that topic. Although I touch on the challenges, it is not my purpose here to convince you that there is a problem. The challenges are followed by doable considerations that can positively improve your life.

In an effort to make it easy for you to find the solutions, the highlighted word **consider** under each topic indicates where the solutions begin. The solutions continue until the next topic begins. If you don't want to read about the challenge—just skip to the word **consider** and check out the solutions. I realize that the number of considerations may be overwhelming—or at least it was to me when I was writing them. Start by considering just one thing and incorporate that into your life—switch to a chemical free laundry detergent, toss your toxic air fresheners or declutter a drawer. Then consider another solution. Before you know it you will be incorporating a few solutions from each chapter. It has taken over 55 years for us to integrate 80,000 chemicals into our lives and it will surely take us many more to eliminate them. Remember, considering is the first step to healing. Think about healing one consideration at a time. As Josh Billings, author of the Farmers Almanac said, be like a postage stamp and stick to one thing until you get there.

Instead of blaming yourself for feeling guilty or ignorant about these issues, consider the positive impact of your contribution to the solution. Assuredly, the subject matter is negative but the suggested solutions are positive. If you can not relate to a topic, turn the page and find one that inspires you to take action. Stay focused on the positive—the incredible dream of a sustainable world in harmony with nature. Always remember, you matter!

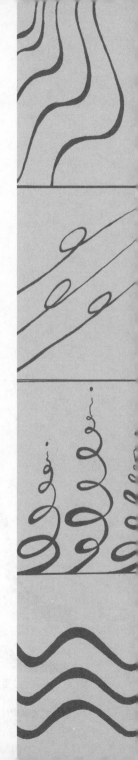

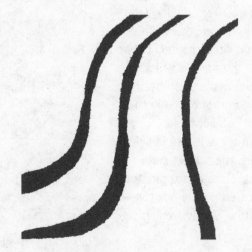

EARTH

Chapter 2

In This Chapter —✦— Products and practices relating to the home, office or land

Introduction to Earth

Lying on the river bank, far away from man-made intrusions, I look up at the star-laden sky and am reminded of the magnificence of our universe. I feel connected to the life force that is present in nature. This beautiful place, a gift from nature, motivates me to continue creating essential environments.

Although I cannot *see* any chemicals, I know that even in this beautiful place, they have infiltrated the river, the land, the air and my body. Imagine all of us living on one long river. Everything that we do goes into that river and flows on to someone else. We and everything on this earth are intrinsically interrelated. This chapter will help you to maintain a clean and safe river at your riverbank and for all of us who are downstream.

In this chapter, you will discover easy solutions for creating an essential environment associated with the materials and products in your life in the categories of: Home Accessories, Home Maintenance, Materials & Components, Office, Outdoor, Personal Care, Pet Care and Travel. Discover how simple it is to make better choices toward healing your world.

Traveling along the highway one day, I saw a ten-story building off in the distance. The fact that it did not have any windows sparked my interest. As I drove closer, the sign on the top of the building became clear—Personal Storage. What an icon for our consuming times. We now have so much "baggage" that we need to construct ten-story concrete buildings to contain our stuff. Baggage or clutter is one of the largest obstacles to blocking your path to an essential environment and better health. In the section under Clutter, you will learn how to clear your excess baggage to unblock and unclog your life. It is possible and you are capable of stopping the flow of excess stuff that depletes your resources and your energy. Removing this clutter affords us the opportunity to gain clarity in our thinking, our lives and our environment.

One house creates more pollution each year than one vehicle. Over 100 chemical pollutants from household products end up in sewage systems. Our homes contain countless chemicals that are harmful to our health. Are you feeling depressed or tired, suffering from allergies or asthma? Chances are that something in your environment may be causing this dis-ease. The chemicals in household materials, from carpeting to paints, fragrances to scented candles, can hinder your ability to sustain optimal health.

Your health is greatly affected by the environments in which you inhabit. Harmony and balance, important factors in supporting your health, are created when spaces are authentic and sustainable. Using natural colors that are found in nature and materials that complement the setting create authenticity in a structure. For example, a Tudor style home does not look authentic in a farm setting, just like a log cabin does not look authentic on an urban street. Your environment should be complementary and compatible with its surroundings and the flow of nature. Sustainability, another important factor for health, relies on using products and practices that maintain, not deplete biological resources. Regrettably, in the world today we manufacture approximately 100 million types of products and *not one* of them is 100 percent sustainable.

When incorporating the following suggestions into your life, try to understand that each individual person, fabric, or material has the potential to react differently to a particular suggested use. Before you begin, it is recommended that you read the directions carefully and remember to test any new products first. Call or visit your physician or other health care provider should you have any health care-related questions or concerns about creating an essential environment.

Take the next step toward experiencing the joy of living with an appreciation of and connection to your surroundings.

Considerations for Earth

With the average person moving 11.7 times in the course of his or her lifetime, a conscious connection to the land and the flow of nature is indispensable now more than ever. This chapter helps you to take the next step toward experiencing the joy of living with an appreciation of and connection to your surroundings—without harmful chemicals.

Home Accessories

APPLIANCES

Many of our daily activities revolve around the appliances and equipment in our homes such as stoves, refrigerators, vacuum cleaners, televisions and computers.

The Environmental Protection Agency (EPA) created the label, Energy Star, for products that meet strict energy- and water-efficient criteria. The Energy Star label makes it easy for you to recognize the most efficient models.

Appliances that are energy-efficient sometimes can cost a little extra. However, the initial costs will certainly be offset by the increased savings on your energy bill and the decreased emissions will better support your health.

► **Consider** the transformation that could occur if just one in ten homes used Energy Star qualified appliances. It would be like planting 1.7 million acres of new trees. What a wonderful choice to make.

Your utility bill can be reduced with Energy Star appliances. More than 35 different categories of Energy Star appliances are available from which to choose. Water-Efficient Appliances are discussed in the Water chapter.

Using a gas- or electric-powered stove is a personal choice. If you are sensitive to chemicals, choose an electric stove as even the slightest fumes from a gas stove may be adding to your dis-ease.

When shopping for a vacuum cleaner, choose one with a High Efficiency Particulate Air (HEPA) filter to collect smaller airborne particles as you clean.

There are alternatives to preparing food with your microwave oven. There have been very few scientific studies on the effects to the human body from eating microwaved foods even though they have been in use for decades. This is not surprising as the small appliance industry and their lobbyists wield a lot of power. How many would they sell if it were called a radiation oven? Whether or not microwaves are harmful, can cause cancer, alter food nutrients or cause digestive disorders is not my concern here. The fact remains that the controversy over the risks of using a microwave oven exists. Why would I want my food to be nuked or zapped when I can cook it conventionally just as easily with a little planning and a lot less risk? Using a toaster oven can be just as easy for reheating or warming food.

ARTS & CRAFTS

From professional artists to children's scribbling, the creative process can be toxic as a result of the fumes generated by the materials and medium selected. Paints, turpentine, glues, paper, markers, solder, ink, dyes, wax, crayons, chalk and chemical sprays are a few of the materials that can be toxic.

► **Consider** substituting human- and earth-friendly materials when possible, especially for children. Make sure the creative process takes place in a well ventilated space. Wear protective gloves, goggles, aprons and clothing when the chance of coming in contact with harmful chemicals is present.

Non-toxic paints, glues, crayons and recycled paper are available today for safe, eco-friendly arts and crafts. Your creativity will be enhanced and supported by using these products.

BED LINENS, BLANKETS & TOWELS

If you are having trouble sleeping or if you are bothered by allergies or asthma, these maladies could be side effects from your sensitivity to your bed linens and bath towels. You spend one-third of your life sleeping, a fact that highlights the value of creating an essential environment in and around your bed.

Synthetic blended sheets and no-iron cotton sheets are usually covered with a permanent press formaldehyde resin. Sounds lovely, does it not? Symptoms of exposure to formaldehyde include headaches, rashes, nausea, watery eyes and a scratchy throat. Wrinkle-resistant and no-iron fabrics are also treated with formaldehyde.

Man-made fibers such as polyester, acrylic and synthetic blended fabrics contain petroleum and other chemicals that can emit gases as you sleep. Even conventionally grown cotton can be toxic since it absorbs 25 percent of the pesticides applied worldwide.

Your bed clothes should promote comfort and sweet dreams, not allergic reactions and nightmares.

▶ **Consider** that it is important to use natural fibers such as cotton, linen, silk, wool and hemp for your bed linens, towels and blankets. These fabrics are pleasant to your skin and allow your bed to breathe. Certified organic cotton is produced without chemicals and eco-friendly green cotton is processed with lower-impact chemicals than conventional cotton. One hundred percent cotton sheets, towels and blankets are sold in most bed and bath stores. Always wash fabrics and towels in free-and-clear laundry detergent as an additional way to keep the chemicals out of your bedroom. Your bed clothes should promote comfort and sweet dreams, not allergic reactions and nightmares.

CUT FLOWERS

Almost everybody loves flowers. In February alone, Americans buy 100 million roses. Unfortunately, they are not organic. I was shocked to learn that floriculture consumes more deadly chemicals than any other segment of agriculture. Fortunately, we do not eat these flowers, but laborers who tend to these crops are at extreme risk working in confined greenhouses with toxic chemicals.

Most of the flowers sold in the U.S. are imported from South America where pesticide regulations and safety laws for farm workers are not as stringent or perhaps nonexistent.

Providing bug-free flowers that pass inspection forces flower growers to use approximately 650 gallons per acre of extremely dangerous chemicals including neurotoxins and carcinogens. Even domestic flower farms use huge amounts of carcinogenic chemicals in their growing methods. Air, water and floral workers have been heavily contaminated. To add to this tragic scenario, more than 4 trillion cut flowers sold last year in the U.S. were genetically-engineered. A rose is *not* a rose when chemicals are added.

Other products such as plant shine sprays and those promising to remove dust from plastic flowers, are usually chemicals in aerosol cans. Avoid them.

▶ **Consider** that every time you buy cut flowers, you are supporting these toxic practices and bringing unwanted chemicals into your space. The good news is that Organic Bouquet is the first national distributor that is now selling organic flowers. Organic flowers are certified the same way as organic produce and are grown without harmful chemicals. Your local stores, restaurants, florists, schools and businesses can obtain organic flowers by calling 877-899-2468 or by going to www.organicbouquet.com. Whole Foods Markets, Wild Oats Markets and other health food stores also sell organic flowers. They can also be purchased in-season from your local farmers' markets and of course you can always grow your own.

For longer enjoyment of your organic cut flowers, put a drop of free and clear dish detergent in the water and refresh daily.

To keep your house plants clean and sparkling, wipe the leaves with a very mild solution of free and clear dish detergent and water. Avoid dried flowers as they are dust catchers.

DISHES & TABLEWARE

In our fast paced, fast-food culture, the topic of setting a table may seem outdated. Plastic ware, paper plates and throw away napkins have crept into our lives unnoticed.

▶ **Consider** that our disposable dinnerware adds to the pollution of your essential environment. Glass, ceramic, pottery, stoneware and stainless steel represent all of the words we like—sustainable, reusable, refillable, and washable. I take that back, perhaps you do not like the word washable. In that case, you need a pep talk here. Remember the words of Mahatma Gandhi, "You must be the change you wish to see in the world." Use reusable dishes and tableware for an eco-friendly choice.

FURNITURE

Purchasing furniture is often a major investment. Just like so many other products we buy, furniture has a life cycle. The life cycle involves resources, packaging, transportation, maintenance, refurbishing or recycling and disposal. The cycle can either be safe and life sustaining or toxic and wasteful. Purchasing home or office furniture is no different.

▶ **Consider** that "green" furniture manufacturers are supporting the life cycle of their products by embracing safe, sustainable-harvested materials, packaging products to minimize waste and offering ways to reuse, recycle and recover furniture.

When purchasing furniture, use the 4 Rs of responsible purchasing for a sustainable environment—reduce, reuse, recycle and recover. Ask the manufacturer which resources are used, what are their packaging and distribution practices, and how can the furniture be disposed of in the future. When we all start asking, someone will eventually hear us. (See Sources.)

MATTRESSES & PILLOWS

Nearly all mattresses are manufactured with crude oil and natural gases. Check the mattress label and it will probably list polyurethane, foam, styrofoam, nylon and polyester. These materials are derived from petroleum which is very conveniently not mentioned on the label. Nor does the label state that the mattress is treated with fire retardants, microbial and fabric processing that are better known as harmful chemicals. Sometimes the sizing material used to weave the textiles utilizes polyvinyl alcohol (PVA) in its manufacturing. The insulation material is comprised of formaldehyde soaked cardboard. These plastics, foams and polyesters *all* emit toxic gases.

Some organic mattresses and pillows may be masquerading as natural when in actuality their organic fabric is sprayed with chemicals after the certification has been received. The term "certified organic" cotton or wool refers only to the growing process. In short, mattresses and pillows may be labeled as certified organic without having to divulge the final chemical application that completes the process. Ask questions. Remember the manufacturing process is not over until it is over. What innocently begins as a natural product can be tainted easily and unnoticeably with final touches of dangerous contaminants.

Many mattress producers purchase their cotton and wool from other countries where the certification process often does not meet United States' standards. Wool is another

Use the 4 Rs of responsible purchasing for a sustainable environment— reduce, reuse, recycle and recover.

wonderful fabric that starts out pure and ends up being commercially processed with hydrochloric acid. Luckily, some manufacturers clean their wool with good old fashioned soap and water.

▶ **Consider** that your mattress is an important purchase when it comes to keeping the toxins out of your life. A natural mattress is the key to overall health and can improve sleep, lower back pain, allergies, arthritis and asthma.

Organic and natural mattresses are made with natural rubber cores, steel springs or untreated wood slats. These mattresses are padded with certified organic cotton and chemical-free, naturally flame retardant wool and are biodegradable. Natural 100 percent latex is an option for moisture prone sleeping environments. Ask the manufacturer if any chemicals have been used in the processing and/or the finishing process of your mattress or pillow. This is especially important if you have any chemical sensitivity.

A less expensive alternative to a complete natural mattress set is a removable wool mattress topper. This topper can attain some of the benefits of a natural bed, especially if you put cotton barrier covers on your mattress and box spring to protect it from dust and dust mites.

The variety of materials used in pillows brings to mind a hotel that had a pillow "menu." On the night stand there was a menu listing eight different pillows available for delivery to the room. I gave them high marks for originality, but really, did I need this pressure? It was a classic example where having many choices is more confusing than having a single choice. Down-filled, down-feather-filled, polyester, non-polyester, hypo-allergenic, buckwheat, natural latex and herbal-filled were some of the pillows being offered. After finally deciding what type of pillow to choose, I now had to ponder the choice of soft, medium or firm. When shopping for pillows, the best choice is one that is filled with a natural material such as cotton, down or buckwheat and is covered in organic, untreated cotton. Hypo-allergenic usually means the pillow is made from synthetic materials that do not attract dust mites thereby reducing allergy symptoms. Use cotton pillowcases or coverings that can be washed regularly in chemical-free detergent.

SLEEP

Sleep clinics report that the three leading causes of sleeplessness are alcohol, caffeine and television. Sleep is the way the body repairs itself and just like other mechanical engines, it cannot be fixed while running. Creating an essential environment in your bedroom is the key to getting the proper sleep and letting your engine restore itself. Normally, our bodies are resilient enough to metabolize and eliminate toxins in our environment by natural detoxification, but this has become increasingly difficult due to the excess exposure and bombardment of chemicals that daily invade our spaces. A good night's sleep allows our bodies the necessary downtime to rejuvenate and restore.

▶ **Consider** that when a space is balanced and in harmony, the energy it creates will support the activity you want to achieve. The following suggestions will help you get a good night's sleep: Keep the energy quiet in the bedroom by using calming colors of the earth such as cream, pale yellow or tan. Choose the color of water, pale blue or green, as additional tranquil colors for the bedroom. Use solid color sheets, as they are more calming than patterned ones. Place the head of your bed against a solid wall. Put your bed where your feet are not pointing out of the doorway. While you are sleeping, keep any bathroom and closet doors closed that are in the bedroom. Do not sleep where your body is reflected in a mirror when you lie down making it hard for your subconscious mind to rest. Remove all chemicals and scented products such as candles and potpourri from the bedroom. Make sure images and sounds in your bedroom are calming and supportive. Check for any shadows that cast scary shapes in your child's room as they can cause sleeplessness. Try to establish a regular sleep schedule. Avoid television and strenuous workouts as bedtime since they are not conducive to good sleep habits. Read a few pages of an inspiring book to relax your mind before retiring. Remember that you are creating a safe and comforting haven enabling your body patterns and rhythms to occur in their natural capacity—sleep.

Creating an essential environment in your bedroom is the key to getting the proper sleep.

Home Maintenance

BATTERIES

Disposable batteries enter our lives and exit into our landfills from many different sources. They are costly for you and your environment.

▶ **Consider** that rechargeable batteries are the better choice to reduce waste and save money. There are two kinds of rechargeable batteries.

Nickel-cadmium (Ni-Cad) batteries are the most popular and can be recharged approximately 750 times. Although a better choice than disposable batteries, they *are* made from toxic metals that need to be disposed of properly at hazardous waste facilities.

The other type of rechargeable batteries is nickel metal hydride (NiMH) that is made *without* heavy metals. They have twice the energy of Ni-Cad batteries but generally run for shorter periods and are usually only rechargeable about 400 times. Being both rechargeable and environmentally safe, they provide a better choice for batteries.

CLEANING CLOTHS, SPONGES & PAPER TOWELS

It is easy to see how we can become overwhelmed when we have to be concerned about the kind of sponges and cleaning cloths to purchase. Instead of choosing a certain color or brand, simply aim for the least harmful type available. Most sponges sold in the U.S. contain a synthetic disinfectant, a pesticide known as triclosan. Washing dishes and counter tops with this chemical can cause bacteria to become more resistant over time as well as adding chemicals to your life. Not to mention the added chemicals in your life. The more chemicals we use the less effective they become.

▶ **Consider** avoiding sponges that claim to kill odors or are antibacterial. Pure cotton cloths or pure cellulose sponges are your best choice. When they get dirty, boil them for five minutes to kill the bacteria. They can also be laundered or cleaned in your dishwasher with a load of dishes.

Micro-fiber cloths contain up to 80 percent polyester and 20 percent polyamide. These cloths can be used with ecologically safe products but the fact remains that chemicals are used to produce them. Feather dusters stir up and move more dust then they collect. Using a slightly damp, cotton terry cloth rag is a better choice.

Paper towels are an easy, sanitary way to clean up messes, but they are costly to you and the environment. Use cotton towels that can be laundered and reused. When and if you do use paper towels, buy recycled products and make sure they are not bleached with chlorine which can create dioxins that are easily transferred to your skin and food. These free and clear paper towels; free of fragrances, chemicals and dyes, can be recycled in your compost pile.

CLEANING PRODUCTS & EQUIPMENT

Here is an area that will allow you can make a huge difference in your world. The majority of cleaning products used today are filled with chemicals that can rob you of your health. We are more apt to take a closer look at our food labels than our cleaning products, yet the ingredients in our cleaning products are just as important relative to your good health.

We have let marketers of these products lull us into thinking that we need a special product or a powerful industrialized chemical solution for every household cleaning chore. Tally the number of cleaners from your garage to your kitchen sink, from your laundry to your bathroom, and I am sure you will understand what I mean.

▶ **Consider** supporting your well-being while supporting a great company; Seventh Generation, Inc. is the leading brand of non-toxic and environmentally safe household products. I am always impressed and refreshed by their human- and eco-friendly "corporate" mindset. Their name is derived from the Iroquois belief that "In our every deliberation, we must consider the impact of our decisions on the next seven generations." Every time you use a Seventh Generation product, you are making a difference by saving natural resources, reducing pollution, keeping toxic chemicals out of the environment and making the world a safer place for this and the next seven generations. Support this and other companies such as Ecover, Bi-O-Kleen, and Dr. Bronner's that are making a difference in your world. See the Sources for companies and products mentioned here.

You can rid your life of unnecessary chemicals in cleaning products by choosing four basic cleaning ingredients that are time-tested, safe, inexpensive and easy to use: white vinegar, baking soda, borax and Bon Ami. Since making the switch, cleaning my home has become so much easier, healthier and less expensive. Just think of all those bottles of chemical cleaners you will no longer need to stock or use or absorb.

The following are considerations, using chemical-free products and eco-friendly practices, when cleaning:

Since making the switch, cleaning my home has become so much easier, healthier and less expensive.

General cleaning. Most surfaces are easily cleaned with a solution of half white vinegar and half water with a drop of free and clear dish detergent. For a non-toxic cream cleanser, make a paste using baking soda and water. Bon Ami, a natural cleanser comprised of feldspar and calcite, can also be used. Found in most grocery stores, Bon Ami has been used since 1890 as a chlorine-, phosphate-, perfume- and dye-free cleaning product. Use it to polish and clean hard surfaces such as countertops and floors.

Borax is another natural cleaner that has been around for many years. It is a natural occurring mineral compound composed of sodium, boron, oxygen and water. It is great for using in the laundry, but also removes mold and mildew and deodorizes and disinfests. For a free guide for household uses visit www.dialcorp.com.

Additional safe cleaning ingredients include biodegradable, fragrance-free detergent and liquid soap, lemon juice, organic apple cider vinegar and liquid wax jojoba. Substitute these ingredients in place of traditional chemical cleaners. Various applications are listed below.

Bathrooms. Because bathrooms sometimes need that little extra cleaning punch, the choices of products containing harsh chemicals are endless.

▶ **Consider** that all of the same safe cleaning ingredients discussed above can be used in the bathroom. In addition, there are also non-toxic mildew removers and orange oil citrus cleaners that will help with the tough areas in bathrooms.

Carpets. Odors, spots and dirt are a common reason to reach for the traditional carpet cleaner—but stop; they too can contain a combination of harsh chemicals.

▶ **Consider** that safer carpet care products are available that contain no known hazardous ingredients. These products help to remove chemicals in newly installed carpet such as sealed in chemical residue in carpet backing and sealed in chemicals that can emit harmful toxins from petroleum-based carpeting. Safer shampoos and sealants also help to repel stains and dirt.

Vacuuming is the best way to remove the pollutants that have become lodged in your carpeting. A High Efficiency Particulate Air Filter (HEPA) vacuum cleaner is the best way to prevent the captured pollutants from blowing back into the air. Kicking your shoes off at the door can significantly cut down on the dirt and pollutants you need to clean off your floor.

To remove unwanted odors from carpets and rugs, sprinkle a liberal amount of baking soda, cornmeal, salt, white rice or borax over the carpet, wait 20 minutes and vacuum. To spot clean carpets or rugs, use sparkling mineral water or club soda and a drop of free and clear dish detergent. The bubble action and the salt combine to lift out dirt. The sooner you treat a spot, the easier it is to remove.

Dishes & pans. Cancer patients, upon leaving the hospital, are often counseled not to use their dishwashers due to the residue left on the dishes from detergents.

▶ **Consider** using free-and-clear dish detergent that is safe for you, your dishes and your environment. To remove tough stains and food that is stuck to pots and pans, sprinkle a little salt in the pan with some room temperature water. Let the pan sit for an hour or overnight and it will be easy to clean.

Drains. Drain cleaners are in the same category as oven cleaners; they are made of harsh and harmful chemicals.

▶ **Consider** that the first line of defense is to use a plunger to unclog a blocked drain. Next try bacteria-based enzyme cleaners, available at most health food stores, to break down any organic matter.

If these suggestions are ineffective in unclogging the drain, try these home remedies. If water is not backed up in the sink, you can pour a cup of baking soda followed by three cups of boiling water down the drain. Repeat until the drain unclogs. A more powerful method is to pour one cup of baking soda followed by a cup of vinegar and a cup of boiling water down the drain. Cover the drain and let it sit for 15 minutes. Finish by pouring a gallon of boiling water down the drain to flush out the clog. If this fails, call in a professional to make use of a plumber's snake.

As a preventative practice, periodically pour boiling water down the drain to keep it clear. Keep hair and vegetable scraps from going down the drain with a drain cover. Toss your vegetable scraps in the compost instead of the disposal.

Furniture. The smell of most furniture polish sends off alarms in my brain about neurotoxins. A substance called nitrobenzene is commonly used in furniture polish and could be fatal if swallowed.

▶ **Consider** using a solution of a quarter cup of apple cider vinegar or lemon juice with several drops of olive oil or liquid jojoba wax on a soft cloth to polish your furniture instead of the harsh chemicals that may very likely be causing you daily dis-ease.

Glass. Mix a solution of equal parts of white vinegar and water with a drop of free and clear dish detergent to apply on your glass and mirrors. You will find that initially vinegar and water may cause streaks. The streaking is temporary and is due to the

Most laundry detergent, dryer sheets, and fabric softeners contain fragrances, dyes, perfumes and other chemicals that are not skin- or eco-friendly.

wax build up from store-bought window cleaners. Ironically, you might have to clean the chemical cleaners residue away before you reach a real, naturally healthy shine.

▶ **Consider** that once the vinegar and water takes off the wax, the windows and mirrors will be much easier and less non-toxic to clean the next time. Be patient, as it may take several periods of cleaning the surface and a little elbow action to remove the wax.

Laundry. If we spend one-third of our lives sleeping and the remainder awake and dressed, 100 percent of the time our skin is in contact with fabric. Most laundry detergent, dryer sheets, and fabric softeners contain fragrances, dyes, perfumes and other chemicals that are not skin- or eco-friendly. Seventh Generation states on its Natural Laundry Detergent, "If every household in the United States replaced just one bottle of 50 ounce ultra petroleum based liquid laundry detergent with our 50 ounce vegetable based product, we could save 280,000 barrels of oil, enough to heat and cool 16,000 U.S. homes for a year!"

▶ **Consider** using chemical-free detergents (free of perfumes, dyes and harmful chemicals), non-chlorine bleach, borax and white vinegar instead. Companies like Seventh Generation, Ecover, Bi-O-Kleen, and Dr. Bronner provide safe, non-chemical alternatives. (See Sources.)

For a healthy, chemical-free alternative to dryer sheets and fabric softeners, add a cup of white vinegar to the rinse cycle. White vinegar also removes odors. For tough stains, use a dab of safe dishwashing liquid.

Another natural solution for clean laundry is chemical-free ceramic capsules. Two types of activated ceramics ionize water to penetrate fabric and lift out dirt particles without harming the fibers. They are hypo-allergenic and last up to 700 wash loads in a top-loading machine. This sounded too good to be true, so I tried them myself and was thrilled with the results. For clothes that are really soiled, it is best to use the capsules along with the vegetable-based enzyme cleaner that is also available.

Mold. Conventional methods used for killing mold involve chlorine bleach which is not human- or environmentally-friendly.

▶ **Consider** using a less toxic solution of borax and water. Wipe down surfaces in the shower with borax but *do not rinse* as the borax residue will retard mold growth. Two teaspoons of tea tree oil mixed with two cups of water or undiluted white vinegar can also be effective in fighting mold.

Ovens. One solution to harsh oven cleaning chemicals is a self-cleaning oven that cleans with intense heat instead of chemicals.

▶ **Consider** using baking soda and water to clean your oven. Make a watery paste out baking soda and water, spread it on the bottom of the oven and let it set overnight to loosen the baked-on grime. Clean out the oven the next day, treating the tough spots with a little liquid detergent to cut the grease. Rinse the entire residue from the oven.

Silver. Who would not like to have a non-toxic, easy way to polish silver?

▶ **Consider** trying another earth- and human-friendly solution that works and is easy. Fill a sink with 2-3 inches of very hot water. Add and dissolve 1 teaspoon of salt and 1 teaspoon of baking soda. Lay a sheet of aluminum foil in the hot water. Submerge the silver in the sink for 2-3 minutes. Remove silver and wipe away tarnish with a clean cotton cloth. Repeat if necessary. Be careful not to use this method on decorative antique silver knives because the blade may separate from the handle. Another alternative is to use non-abrasive toothpaste instead of silver polish, but then you are back to a labor intensive exercise.

A product called Qwicksilver uses this same concept and also cleans brass, copper, bronze, gold, jewelry and stainless steel. This self-acting electrolytic metal cleaning plate consists of different metals. When placed in a sink with the activator of sodium and soda it removes tarnish from silver, copper, bronze, gold, stainless steel and most brass. It is 100 percent environmentally friendly, biodegradable and the best part—it is self acting.

Cleaning equipment. Eco- and human-friendly cleaning equipment is becoming more and more available; in fact, it is usually sold right alongside the chemical guzzling equipment.

Think of the time, money and space you will save by not having to stock up on chemical-laden products and equipment.

► **Consider** when purchasing cleaning equipment, it supports an essential environment. Vacuum cleaners are discussed in the Air chapter, but using one with a HEPA filter is a better choice. Mop heads and sponges that can be laundered are a better choice than ones that come with chemicals already applied for "easy clean up" and easy chemical consumption.

A handy, ecological piece of cleaning equipment is a vapor steam cleaner. They use water to clean and sanitize almost any household surface and are easy to use. The extra high temperature can kill bacteria, mold and dust mites; remove grease, grime and mildew and deodorize carpets and bedding. A steamer can clean floors, windows, sinks, ovens, stoves, toilets, walls, showers and cribs. Items such as jewelry, grills, outdoor furniture, golf clubs, toys, upholstery, clothing and more can also be cleaned with a steamer. Available in several sizes from canisters to handheld models, steamers are efficient, cost-effective and a perfect solution for keeping cleaning chemicals out of your life.

Overall, cleaning products and equipment can prove to be very safe when accompanied by a little knowledge about how to make better, non-chemical choices. Knowing that you can protect yourself by making better choices in selecting cleaning supplies, think of the time, money and space you will save by not having to stock up on chemical-laden products and equipment.

CLUTTER

Clutter may be the largest block to your optimal health. It is anything you do not use or love—unwanted gifts, outdated magazines, old clothes, broken appliances, and more. Clutter is visual noise that zaps your energy by requiring your attention both consciously and subconsciously. It possesses a subliminal tendency suggesting disorder aesthetically and mentally.

Due to the potential fire hazard of living in paper and wood housing, Asian cultures built concrete sheds to store their valuables. Every season they would bring one object, a painting, a tapestry or a vase, into their dwelling. Appreciating and focusing their attention on just one object for the season created a sense of peace and harmony. In our culture, overabundance has resulted in cluttered environments that cause unfocused attention which contributes to a state of mental and physical disarray.

▶ **Consider** that 80 percent of the stuff we use comes from 20 percent of the stuff we have. Removing the clutter from a space will allow the eye to rest and the mind to be clear. Clearing clutter is essential to manifesting better health and to creating a supportive environment. The beauty of clearing clutter is that it works on unblocking all levels of your life—physical, spiritual, intellectual and emotional. It is similar to detoxifying your visual world.

Just think if all the things in your space had a "home," a designated place, then it would be easier to find, use and replace them. For example, if your scissors and tape have a "home" every time you need them, you would know where they are and where to put them when you are finished using them. Also, when your belongings are easy to access, they are more conducive to use. This saves time and energy for everyone.

Designate a home for each of your belongings. If you do not have enough space, pare down so you no longer have to trip over, push aside, stack up or misplace your life. Sounds like a good time to plan a community yard sale.

Here is a trick for clearing clutter—books, photos, clothing, toxic food, collections, papers, art, equipment, toys and supplies. Touch everything in your life (at least once a year) and consciously label it "yes," "no" or "maybe." Yes means I use and love it, no means I do not use and love it, and maybe means maybe I use and love it. Keep the "yes" items; recycle, discard or give away the "no" items. Set the "maybes" aside. Revisit them in 48 hours and surprisingly you *will* know in which category to place them. If that particular item resonates with your lifestyle at this juncture, you will automatically know where it belongs, even if it belongs somewhere else. It is that easy.

Reduce the clutter coming into your life. Choose to appreciate beautiful things in the store or gallery. You do not have to own every beautiful object that crosses your path to appreciate it. Identify ways clutter enters your life and take action to change, redirect or reduce this flow. For example, if catalogs tend to pile up on the kitchen counter, place a recycle box in the garage or closet to collect them as you organize the daily mail. The key is trusting that your life will be better by letting go of unused and excess stuff. If you hold on to everything, be assured that you will never be successful in locating what is necessary when you need it.

Before buying or acquiring something new, think of the implication it has on your life. Does it require maintaining, dusting, storing, refilling or painting? The consequences of stuff can be time consuming and expensive. Fewer things will give you more time, energy and abundance. Be not afraid of an empty shelf or drawer.

Be not afraid of an empty shelf or drawer.

GARAGES

How does the saying go, "You are where you park?" Garages may be the most noxious of all living spaces. Car fumes, oil, yard equipment, paint, overflowing household clutter and a myriad of cans and bottles containing harmful chemicals can be found in most garages.

▶ **Consider** creating an essential environment in your garage to improve your life.

Start by removing clutter and recycling any toxic chemicals that have piled up. Play music, sing or whistle while you work. Use the "yes, no or maybe" technique under Clutter to rid your life of the other unwanted items. Call a waste collection agency to dispose of old insecticides, herbicides and other toxic materials. Never use or dispose of them yourself. The end result will be a garage that is non-toxic and eco-friendly.

Modern home design directs most people to enter their home from their garage, back or side door. Whatever entrance you use, and hopefully it is your front door, make it a happy, welcoming space. Paint the walls with your favorite colors or hang up a breath-taking landscape or soothing seaside picture. Even in your garage, make your arrival view beautiful, fun and welcoming.

JUNK MAIL & TELEMARKETING

Now onto one of my biggest pet peeves—junk mail. I set out on a personal quest to stop junk mail from entering my life. I failed. After contacting all the sources of junk mail and requesting that my address be removed from their list, you would think that the problem was solved. Unfortunately, since direct mail companies frequently purchase lists from other sources, within a month or two the junk mail was back. I cringe at the waste that arrives in my mailbox daily. The average American receives about 300 catalogs per year which equates to almost 10.8 billion pounds of paper.

▶ **Consider** registering online at www.dmaconsumers.org/cgi/offmailinglistdave to have your address removed from marketer's mailing lists. This free service can significantly cut unwanted junk mail. You can also send a card with your name, address and signature to Mail Preference Service, Direct Marketing Association, Box 643, Carmel, NY 10512 asking them to remove your name and address. In the meantime, keep recycling and shredding the junk mail to use for packing material.

While I am at it—if telemarketers disrupt your essential space, phone technology is available to block these calls. Visit www.donotcall.gov and register your phone number at no charge.

LIGHT POLLUTION, LIGHTING & LIGHT BULBS

Pollution is not usually associated with light, although light pollution is everywhere and continues to escalate. Excess lighting has caused a lightening of our night sky and has made most of our cities fifty times brighter than their surrounding areas. Only 10 percent of Americans can actually see the Milky Way. Counting your lucky stars is becoming more of a challenge.

We spend most of our time inside, either at our workplace or within our homes which makes light quality a vital objective. The proper lighting in appropriate areas can actually brighten up your day in more ways than one. Good lighting can have a positive effect on your personality, attitude, and the inevitable winter blues better known as seasonal affected disorder (SAD). Research has found that lighting has an effect on the rates of achievement in school children.

Lighting has an effect on the rates of achievement in school children.

There are two types of artificial light, outdoor and indoor. Outdoor lighting includes billboards, street lights, parking lot lights, and any façade or landscape lighting. We equate lighting at night with the promotion of safety, security and utility. Poor lighting is responsible for urban sky glow and light trespassing that can create a chaotic frenzy of brightness, wasting energy wattage and money. Most artificial lighting provides illumination equivalent to only 1 or 2 percent of the intensity of daylight.

Artificial and excessive lighting can cause an imbalance in your environment. In an effort to provide better visibility, improper and unnecessary lighting becomes a clear-cut factor in many nighttime accidents caused by blinded or confused drivers and pedestrians. Glare never assists in providing better visibility and light trespassing often offends neighbors. Also, keep in mind that night creatures, such as sea turtles, various species of birds and many insects, require darkness to reproduce and incubate their young.

Incandescent or traditional light bulbs, including halogen are not as efficient, nor are they as long-lasting as compact fluorescent bulbs. Thirty percent of the light which emanates from traditional, incandescent light bulbs is wasted.

▶ **Consider** using only energy-efficient lighting sources and managing the direction of light sources away from areas that do not want or need exposure. Improving the quality and efficiency of your light bulbs will have tremendous impact on your environment.

Compact fluorescent bulbs with electronic ballasts, not magnetic ballasts, use 75 percent less energy than standard bulbs and emit much less carbon dioxide over their approximately 10-year lifetime. Compact fluorescent bulbs come in globe, flood, 100-watt, 60-watt and 3-way replacement models. Install time controls to minimize your impact on glare and wasted energy. Choose models with the Energy Star label, which are guaranteed to last at least 6,000 hours. When choosing night-lights, the blue-glowing, super-efficient electroluminescent lights that use only .04 watts compared with 4 watts are the best choice.

Low pressure sodium (LPS) lamps originated in Europe for producing a large amount of light that is energy efficient. Often used for roadway, industrial and security lighting as the bulbs are monochromatic and are very poor in color retention. They have a long-lasting life and do not attract bugs! Use self-charging solar lights for your outdoor lighting needs where possible.

An important factor in selecting light bulbs is the photobiologic spectra. This is the spectral energy a bulb gives off to simulate natural light in order for the body to function at its peak. Natural light provide a full spectrum of light for optimal health. Natural full spectrum light bulbs are the best way to simulate the crisp, full color and ultraviolet spectrum of natural outdoor light.

Neodymium light bulbs give off a full spectrum color, not the yellowish color usually seen in standard incandescent lighting—up to 90 percent less yellow spectral light. Neodymium is a unique natural element that recreates true daylight. Neodymium light bulbs come in long lasting incandescent, fluorescent, compact fluorescent, halogen, ballasts and low pressure sodium lamps. Neodymium lighting comes in 60 to 150 watt bulbs and flood lights.

Fluorescent lighting, which is the most energy-efficient, has improved over the years and full spectrum fluorescent lights are available for commercial use in place of the standard cool or warm colored tubes. Fluorescent bulbs with magnetic ballasts contain a trace of radioactive material, unlike electronically ballast tubes that do not, which make them a healthier choice.

Seventh Generation states that every year Americans throw away over 1.6 billion standard incandescent bulbs. If every household in the U.S. replaced just *one* standard incandescent bulb with long lasting natural spectrum bulb, we could save 132 million kilowatt hours of energy (used to manufacture the bulbs) and 626,000 cubic feet of landfill space.

PACKAGING

Lily Tomlin once told a story about going to the store to buy a wastebasket. After purchasing the wastebasket, the clerk placed it in a bag. When Lily arrived home, she took the wastebasket out of the bag and put the bag in the wastebasket. After all, there is a reason they call it a "waste" basket. Although funny, this sheds light on a sad scenario and wasteful packaging practices that are clogging up our landfills. One-third of an average landfill is made up of packaging material.

► **Consider** consuming products that are not packaged or that have minimal packaging. Take your own bag when shopping and avoid excess packaging. If you only buy a few items, kindly decline the offer of the store's bag.

Support companies that use eco-friendly packaging. Ask companies to use alternatives to the eco-*un*friendly styrofoam "peanuts." Preferable peanuts are made from corn starch, wood or recycled natural materials. Recycled boxes and recycled, unbleached paper are safer environmental choices. Always reuse and recycle packaging materials.

RECYCLING

To recycle means to use again. Americans throw away 2.5 million plastic bottles every hour. A single quart of motor oil, if disposed of improperly, can contaminate up to 2,000,000 gallons of fresh water. Approximately 130 million wireless phones are discarded annually to landfills where many of them can leach toxic lead, arsenic, and cadmium into our environment. Compact disc covers pollute the environment with a flood of PCBs, dioxins, solvents and toxic metals. The statistics go on and on as does the waste.

► **Consider** that recycling will help to reverse the negative effects of our disposable culture. Recycling is good for the earth and it is good for you. Do it as often and as much as you can—it feels good.

"Pre-cycling" is a way to make more conscientious purchases. Before purchasing an item, ask yourself what resources were used in its production. Buy products that are sustainable, recyclable, reusable and/or refillable. For example, choose a wicker laundry basket instead of a plastic one—one is sustainable, one is not. When available, buy products that are made from recycled products.

Recycling is good for the earth and it is good for you.

Find out the recycling locations and practices in your community. Some practices include recycling plastic bags to grocery stores, oil and anti-freeze to gas stations, six-pack rings and household batteries to schools, eyeglasses to the Lions Club, cell phones to electronic stores and leaves into community composting. (See Sources.) Packaging and other items that are not recycled or recyclable in your community becomes garbage and is wasted.

If we recycle just one-tenth of our newspapers, we could save 25 million trees a year. Recycling metal cans reduces energy by 74 percent, water pollution by 76 percent, solid waste by 95 percent and air pollution by 85 percent. For every recycled glass bottle, we save enough energy to light a 100-watt light bulb for 4 hours. The list of benefits for recycling is endless as are the resources available.

Reuse items. If on occasion you have to resort to using disposable things like plastic ware, they can be washed and reused.

Outdated computers are a great item to recycle, yet the National Safety Council estimates that only 11 percent of discarded computers are recycled. Computers that are not recycled can leach heavy metals into groundwater and pollute the air if incinerated. Overseas, legislation already requires proper recycling and disposal of all computers, but here at home, only a few of the major computer companies have a "take back" program. Wireless phones and smoke detectors that contain radioactive waste also need to be recycled properly. In a world based on the premise of built-in obsolescence, it is imperative that we learn to repair, reuse and recycle appliances and machines.

We applaud the Wild Oats Natural Foods Markets' Deli Departments that are switching from plastic containers to those made from 100 percent non GMO corn. When the used containers are returned to the store; they have a special way of composting them in about 40 days. Good job, hope abounds.

The United States Department of Energy estimates that at least 500 million and as many as 3 billion tires are stockpiled in America. There are an additional 270 million tires discarded every year. The good news is that rubber tires are beginning to be recycled into sidewalks by U.S. Rubber Recycling. However, the initial cost is higher than concrete, yet the rubber sidewalks last much longer. As the demand for this new technology increases, commercial and home applications will be discovered such as garden mulch made from tires.

Nike's Reuse-a-Shoe program is an excellent example of earth-conscious recycling programs. Since 1993, this program has recycled all brands of worn-out athletic shoes into materials used in sporting events' surfaces, sidewalks, playgrounds, tracks and courts. NikeReuseAShoe.com. lists stores that accept donations of all brands of athletic footwear.

If you would like to recycle your running shoes that are in good condition, they can be donated to the Shoes for Africa program. Shoes are sent to athletes who are training in West Africa. Visit www.ShoesForAfrica.com

Additional ways to help the environment are to use matches or refillable lighters instead of disposable lighters. Snip the circles of plastic six-pack holders prior to recycling so they are not a hazard to animals. Return unused pharmaceutical drugs, used needles and aspirators to your pharmacist for proper recycling.

Buy in bulk or large size. For example, purchase a large container of shampoo and use it to refill smaller containers. Every one of your baby steps helps.

The architecture and construction of our living spaces has been slower to evolve than our consciousness and lifestyles.

REPAIRS

This may be obvious to some, but look around your environments and see if anything needs to be repaired. Things like door knobs that stick, hinges that are falling off, cracked windows, broken furniture, burned out lamps and equipment that does not work. Just like clutter, items in your environment that are in disrepair take vital energy from you.

▶ **Consider** repairing and restoring all of your personal items to good working condition to allow your life to run smoothly. It can be therapeutic as well as a cost saver in terms of unnecessary expenditures.

SMOKE DETECTORS

Ionization smoke detectors contain radioactive materials on a film coated with americium 241. Although the risk of radiation exposure from these smoke detectors is low, they contain radioactive materials and emit gamma radiation which is a by-product of nuclear power. Due to the content of radioactive materials, ionization smoke detectors are required to be returned to the supplier for disposal. Do not dispose of them with household refuse.

Smoke detectors perform a life saving function in the case of a fire. However, it is reported that smoke detectors in more than 30 percent of residences do not operate properly or have dead or missing batteries.

▶ **Consider** testing your smoke detector and replacing batteries when needed. If possible, your smoke detector can be directly hard-wired to your home AC power. If you hard-wire your detector, use a model that has a battery backup in case of a power outage. Instead of ionizing smoke detectors, choose photoelectric smoke detectors that are free of radioactive materials and that contribute to your gamma-, radiation-free environment.

TIRES

Tired of tires being everywhere but where they belong? Well, believe it or not, tires can actually help fight the battle against pollution. Safety is a tire's most vital attribute. Surprisingly, while improving the handling of your vehicle, ecologically friendly tires also serve as a hidden benefit in fuel economy and waste control.

Specially engineered tires have improved tread wear which depletes fewer raw materials and reduces the collection of discarded tires. Lower rolling resistance in the new design requires less fuel.

This newly designed tire, available at any major automotive company, is the direct descendent of the radial tire introduced in the late 1970s. In fact, the combination of improved rolling resistance and longer lasting tires that utilize silica in production has culminated in a reduction of more than two million gallons of oil. It has also reduced the new tire population by 225 million tires per year and the naturally accompanying scrap tires as well.

▶ **Consider** taking better care of your tires to ensure longevity and top performance. Try to purchase tires that will save money and emissions on the long haul. Check your tire pressure once a month and adjust accordingly. Have your alignment checked periodically and rotate your tires every 6000 miles or so. Finally, make sure to check your tires' tread for uneven wear and signs of damage. These simple considerations can save your life and the life of the tires.

Today, the recycling of tires has significantly increased to nearly 80 percent worldwide. Even so, old tire piles attract mosquitoes, are a fire hazard and release toxins into the air and water when burned. Avoid storing tires because they are a notorious fire risk and produce germ factories. Recycling tires is one alternative for worn-out tires or have them retreaded, if possible. Many wonderful end products are created from recycled tires.

Materials & Components

BUILDING MATERIALS

The architecture and construction of our living spaces has been slower to evolve than our consciousness and lifestyles—sort of like the fashions on Star Trek—their minds have expanded but they are still wearing what appears to be restrictive clothing. Home design is stuck in an old paradigm that does not resonate with our lifestyle or an ecological mindset. It is evolving, but very, very slowly. For example, we have bigger and more auspicious front entrances, yet we elect to enter our homes through our garages.

Materials used in building fall into two categories, man-made and nature-made. Generally man-made materials are more toxic, less sustainable, less expensive and more convenient whereas nature-made materials are not.

Similar to purchasing organic vegetables versus the standard fare, the cost of man-made materials never factors in the associated and accumulated cost of pollution and disposal of toxic substances.

Toxic materials of specific concern to your health include pressure-treated wood that is treated with arsenic (check your child's swing set or your deck) and vinyl (polyvinyl chloride—PVC) used in siding, replacement windows and flooring that contain a caustic array of chemicals that never stop releasing toxins.

The ultimate goal in creating essential environments is to use materials that support your good health.

▶ **Consider** that the ultimate goal in creating essential environments is to use materials that support your good health and sustain our planet. To be responsible stewards of our environment, we need to examine the entire cycle of materials used in building or remodeling. Today, thanks to consumer demand, there is a great deal of energetic work being done to provide non-toxic building materials.

Some of those materials include sustainable-forested and salvaged lumber, fiberglass insulation, non-toxic VOC-free paints and solvents, natural linoleum and cork flooring, formaldehyde-free wall and ceiling panels, solar water heaters, energy-efficient lighting, recycled steel and aluminum and recycled rubber used in sidewalks. Volumes have been written recently about "green" building using chemical-free materials and energy-efficient technology. (See Sources.)

If you have the opportunity to make structural changes to your space or are creating a new space, incorporate earth- and human-friendly systems into your plans, such as ground water collection systems, gray water treatment systems, recycling centers and ozone or ultra-violet light treatment for hot tubs and pools. The savings to your health will certainly be worth the investment not to mention your peace of mind.

CARPETS & FLOORING

Most carpeting and rugs are prepared with chemicals and synthetic materials that are derived from crude oil and natural gas. Carpets can hold mold, dirt and dust mites. The dyes, synthetic backing, fire retardants, anti-static and stain-resistant chemicals and glues used in carpeting can cause allergic reactions that have been linked to chemical sensitivity disorders. Newly installed carpet releases these toxic chemicals into your indoor air actively for three months and, although not as active, can continue for much longer. Hardwood floors retain fewer odors than carpets but they are not always feasible.

If you must have carpet, use natural fibers such as 100 percent wool, cotton or hemp that are made with natural dyes. Keep in mind, though, that even these materials are not as clean and green as sustainable wood or other natural flooring materials.

▶ **Consider** using safe flooring that does not add toxicity to your environment such as responsibly harvested and sustainable hardwoods or reclaimed lumber, sisal, coir fiber, bamboo, recycled glass tile, natural stone, ceramic tiles, cork, and natural linoleum. Marmoleum is natural linoleum, allergen-free, biodegradable flooring made from flax resins and wood flour. It comes in 100 cool colors. Hmm, makes you want to redecorate!

If possible, after installing carpet, crack the windows and turn up the heat for 24 hours and stay out of the space. This will help to remove most of the toxic gas out of the carpet. Other solutions include using an ozonation machine or air purifying absorption. (See Air Filtration.)

If you are stuck with synthetic carpet, you can always throw natural fiber rugs over them. They will not block the fumes but will feel better under your feet. To further reduce exposure, wear cotton socks when walking on synthetic carpet. Be sure to protect babies from these toxins on the floor by covering an area with a natural fabric rug. You do not have to sacrifice your health to enjoy that indescribable sensation of walking barefoot on a soft carpet.

Programs backed by the EPA are advocating the recycling of carpets. With an estimated 4.7 billion pounds of carpet being discarded annually, this is a huge environmental issue. Options such as recycled carpets and leased carpets are available.

CEILINGS

Popcorn or textured ceilings collect dust and can easily exacerbate allergies.

▶ **Consider** that this may be a source of allergens if you suffer from allergies. If the ceiling does not contain asbestos or lead paint, one option is to smooth the ceiling by sanding it. If the ceiling contains asbestos or lead, call a professional to assess your situation and your options.

CHEMICAL POLLUTANTS

Fifty countries have endorsed an international agreement banning 12 of the most notorious and persistent pesticides and chemicals. However, the United States is not one of them.

The top six hazardous pollutants and toxic substances are Lead, DEHP, Hexavalent Chromium, Penta BDE, Perchlorethylene and Trichloroethylene (TCE). They are, unfortunately, used in manufacturing products that most of us are exposed to daily.

Although it is nearly impossible to remove all of them, being aware of where and how they exist will help you make better choices in reducing your contact with them.

The most important preventive measure we can take is to conserve and rethink.

Lead is present in paint that was produced and applied prior to 1978 and also in bathtubs that were manufactured prior to 1984.

DEHP is a harmful chemical that makes PVC pliable.

Hexavalent Chromium is used primarily in chrome plating, manufacturing of dyes and pigments, leather tanning and wood preserving.

Penta BDE is used as a flame retardant in textiles, furniture, automobiles, and electric appliances.

Perchlorethylene is used in dry cleaning although many cleaners have removed it from their processing. It is also found in some household products, metal finishes, paint removers, printing inks, adhesives, paper coatings, leather coatings and aerosol sprays.

Trichloroethylene (TCE) is found in some rug cleaners, paint strippers, spot removers, auto cleaning products and typewriter correction fluid.

▶ **Consider** that there are some companies and industries working to stop the use of these chemicals in manufacturing. Be aware, read labels and ask questions about how your products are created and produced and what they contain.

ENERGY

Currently, our primary sources of energy, coal, natural gas, oil, hydro and nuclear power, are not sustainable and do not contribute to a cleaner environment. Most of our current industries and technologies have been developed according to a template that is fashioned for the use of fossil fuels. As a result 68 percent of the electricity used in the United States comes from burning polluted fossil fuels. However, amid all of this prosperity and progress is the undeniable fact that fossil fuels are damaging to the earth's environment. When these fuels are burned, tons and tons of pollution is released into the atmosphere. Fossil fuel extraction also causes destruction to our ecosystems.

A crucial factor in our economy, fossil fuels, are, without a doubt, deeply incorporated into our society with the issue of transportation being slightly more complicated and challenging. Energy is needed for practically everything we touch, from turning up the heat to turning on the light to turning on the television.

Many alternatives loom on the horizon of hope. For transportation, hydrogen and natural gas are being tested due to their ability to greatly reduce harmful emissions. Hybrid technology, electric and gasoline combined engines, are also being introduced for the same reason. Solar energy is slowly becoming more main-streamed and cost effective as a renewable energy source. Wind and biomass energy, organic matter that is converted to energy, continue to emerge as alternative energy sources. To be environmentally successful, hydro (water generated) power technology must be refined so that it ceases to disrupt fish movement, whereas nuclear energy requires reliable and proper disposal of waste.

Another clean, renewable energy source is geothermal heat that relies on underground steam to pull heat up into a building via heat pumps. This energy source can heat a home in the cooler months and cool a home in the warmer months. Some contractors are starting to incorporate it in buildings which will help to mainstream this type of sustainable energy where applicable.

▶ **Consider** that energy efficiency is the quickest, cheapest and cleanest way to extend our world energy supply. The most important preventive measure we can take is to conserve and rethink. Energy is defined as a force, vigor and a capacity. We, *ourselves,* are energy! When you are lacking energy, you try to be efficient while conserving and recharging.

The key word here is efficiency. Efficiently heating, cooling and lighting a space saves money and resources. To accomplish this, the proper equipment, fixtures and light bulbs are needed. The space also needs to be sealed enough to retain the desired temperature or properly ventilated to allow fresh air to do the job.

Many states are opening their electric markets to competition and more than a dozen companies are marketing green power directly to customers. Visit the Department of Energy's Green Power Network website at eren.doc.gov/greenpower or the Green-e Company at www.green-e.org to determine the green power options in your state. Then, with one phone call to your utility or the green utility provider, you can make the switch. This is such a simple thing that each of us can do to conserve energy.

Other considerations for conserving energy include:

- *Replace or clean furnace, air-conditioning and heat-pump filters regularly.*
- *Turn down the temperature of water heaters to warm or 120 degrees.*
- *Insulate your water heater with an insulating blanket.*
- *As they wear out, replace water heaters with "tankless" water heaters.*
- *Use energy-efficient appliances—see www.energystar.gov.*
- *Choose a clean power supplier. Look for the Green-e endorsed companies that provide electricity in your area (www.green-e.org). They draw a significant portion of the power from less toxic, more renewable energy sources, such as wind, sun, biomass and geothermal energy and they do not use nuclear power.*
- *Visit The Department of Energy's Green Power Network (www.eren.doe.gov/greenpower) for green energy options.*
- *Investigate the use of solar power to supplement your home or office energy.*
- *Use self-charging solar lighting for outside areas.*
- *Clean refrigerator coils twice a year.*
- *Recycle old refrigerators as they are an energy drain.*
- *Use low-flow shower heads and faucets.*
- *Turn off lights and appliances when not in use.*
- *Install timers or motion sensors on devices that should not run all the time.*
- *Caulk leaky windows and apply reflective film to windows facing west.*
- *Replace incandescent light bulbs with compact fluorescent bulbs.*
- *Dine by non-toxic candlelight once a week. Make sure to crack a window as candles deplete your oxygen. (See Candles in the Air Chapter.)*
- *Cover the surface of heated water beds to retain as much of the heat as possible.*
- *Insulate water pipes and ducts wherever possible and especially in unheated areas.*

- *Close shades and blinds at night to reduce heat gain or heat loss through windows.*
- *Insulate roofs and exterior walls with dry-blown cellulose or contact a professional contractor to assess your insulation's efficiency.*
- *Replace old, leaky windows with energy-efficient models that have weather stripping, double paned, low-e (low-emittance) glass.*
- *Put low-e film on windows that receive direct sun light. It reflects the heat in summer and retains it in the winter. It is tricky to apply yourself, so you might want to call a professional.*
- *Install a clock thermostat to automatically turn your thermostat down at night.*
- *Plant energy-efficient trees on the south and west side of your building. Well-placed trees and plants can cut the need for air-conditioning and heating.*
- *Enable the energy-saving feature on computers and, when possible, turn them off when not in use.*
- *Use a toaster oven whenever possible instead of a larger oven.*
- *Gas dryers use less energy than electric dryers.*
- *For better efficiency, clean the lint traps in your dryer after each use.*

The necessary technologies do exist to rid us of our energy dependence and the ensuing destruction of fossil fuels. We just need to apply *our energy* to constructive versus destructive methods and practices of creating energy. For a healthier economy, cleaner environment and energy security, you and I have the *power* to make a difference!

PAINTS, SOLVENTS & SEALERS

Paints, lacquers and varnishes that contain chemicals distinctly affect our environment and our health. For the most part, people are completely unaware of the bulk of painted surfaces and objects that they come in contact with in their homes, at workplaces, hospitals, schools, stores and even recreational facilities. There are about 15,000 chemicals that can be used to manufacture paints. These paint products house the potential for serious ecological harm, toxicological risks during production, manufacturing, application, use and the final disposal.

Without exception, *all* of the traditional paint brands available contain very high levels of Volatile Organic Compounds (VOCs). The EPA has confirmed that these VOCs harbor serious health implications such as eye and respiratory tract irritation, headaches, dizziness, visual disorders and visual impairment. Lower levels are capable of affecting the brain, nervous system, blood cells and kidneys. Newly painted rooms can reach contamination levels that are elevated 1000 times higher than outdoor air.

Lead has long been recognized as a dangerous environmental pollutant. Lead was banned from paint in 1978. Old lead paint can create a major amount of exposure when it is not properly removed from surfaces. The scraping and sanding used in removal can cause airborne lead particles to be released and tracked into other parts of your environment, let alone being breathed in unknowingly.

Homes built before 1978 have paint that contains high levels of lead-based paint. Federal law requires that buyers and sellers be informed of lead-based paints before buying, renovating or renting pre-1978 housing. Both unborn babies and young children are severely affected by exposure to lead. Lead, which affects the entire body, can cause convulsions, coma and even death. Long-term exposure to these compounds can lead to cancer.

Most commercial strippers and sealants are made of chemicals that outgas toxic fumes and hazardous odors. The chemicals in paint strippers can cause cancers and birth defects. Coal-tar, a known carcinogen, is the base for most driveway and roof sealants.

▶ **Consider** using a new generation paint that does not emit any solvent vapors into the air and uses regenerative raw materials for binding properties. As a result of the long list of health implications, environmental regulation and consumer demand, new paints and finishers have been developed that are low-VOC or zero VOC *and* lead free. If you have lead paint in your home, investigate having it safely removed by someone who understands the hazards involved. Make sure they know how to dispose of the remaining debris appropriately.

Paints called milk paints are so environmentally friendly that you can pour them into your garden without fear of pollution. Low odor, low or no VOC paints, such as Devoe Paint Wonder Pure and Glidden 2000 are available at most local paint stores. These paints are healthier for you and the environment. Furthermore, recycled paint is available commercially in a range of colors. (See Sources.)

Regrettably, there are no safe paint strippers, only safer ones. There are greener options, such as 3Ms Safest Stripper, Dumond Chemical's Peel Away #6, Easy Off by Klean Strip,and biodegradable Strypeeze by The Savogran Company. (See Sources.)

Safecoat makes paint and several sealers for decks, roofs, concrete, wood, asphalt and multi-purpose use that are less-toxic choices for preventing offensive solvents,

Paints called milk paints are so environmentally friendly that you can pour them into your garden without fear of pollution.

fumes and odors. The good news is that they are great for the earth and for those that have chemical sensitivities. The bad news is that they are usually more expensive than the toxic brands and are available at fewer dealers. Do not dismay, it is worth the expense and the effort.

John Bower of the Healthy House Institute says, "one of the healthiest ways to have a piece of furniture or molding stripped is to take it to a commercial stripper and let them do it. They typically use more powerful products that act quickly, and they have the proper facilities, the correct safety equipment, and an environmentally approved means of disposing of the old finish and spent stripping chemicals. Because some of the healthier strippers are expensive, it may not cost much more to leave the job to a professional."

There are clearly better environmental choices for paint, solvents and sealers but they are not perfect, so precautions are generally in order.

PLASTICS

Plastics which are derived from petroleum have fueled a petroleum-addicted society. Let me highlight a few phrases that I found describing plastic—toxic, outgases volatile organic compounds, lethal, environmental burden, health risks, non-biodegradable, noxious and harmful to ingest—and that about sums it up.

The most toxic plastic is polyvinyl chloride (PVC), commonly known as vinyl. Vinyl chloride, the chemical used to make PVC, is a known human carcinogen. PVC never stops outgassing volatile organic compounds—ever. For instance, PVC products such as vinyl flooring can release chemical softeners called phthalates. PVC flooring has been associated with increases in asthma. Lead additives in PVC mini-blinds were found to cause lead poisoning in some children. Plumbers have also complained about toxic glues used to fit PVC pipes, while some studies suggest that toxic chemicals can leach out of PVC pipes.

Of the estimated 10 billion tons of PVC produced annually in the United States, 60 percent is utilized in building materials such as pipes, siding, windows, flooring, vinyl wall coverings, and window blinds because it is inexpensive and easy to use and replace. While it initially appears to be an ideal material, it carries a high risk to consumers and to the environment.

Twenty percent is used in packaging—including food packaging. The remaining 20 percent is used in hundreds of other products, such as toys, teething rings and rattles, shower curtains, raincoats, garden furniture, medical devices, compact discs, car trim and interiors, office furniture, folders and pens. Surprisingly, in almost every case of implementation, alternatives for PVC use actually do exist.

Our neighbors in Europe are aggressively phasing out PVC—especially in children's clothing. Sony-Europe has a PVC-free packaging policy. Several hospitals overseas are going completely PVC-free. Evian phased out PVC in their plastic containers. Meanwhile in the United States, where the largest amount of PVC is produced, discussions of phasing out and long-term planning are noticeably lacking. We are at an extreme danger level while our government remains stagnated in the infancy stages of actual response.

Telling you to avoid plastic would be like telling you to avoid breathing. But, there *are* a lot of things that you can do to reduce your exposure.

> ▶ **Consider** removing and keeping as much plastic and vinyl products out of your space as possible. Read labels and buy non-PVC materials. When purchasing products, look at the three-arrow triangle recycling symbol—if a V or a 3 is inside a triangle, it is vinyl. It also may be stamped PVC. Read labels and avoid products using chemicals that have *chloro*, *fluor* and *brom* as part of their name.

When making purchases from children's toys to bottled water, flooring, wall coverings and others, select products that are not plastic or do not contain vinyl plastics. Always ask yourself if a better human, eco-friendly version is available. Avoid plastic plates, utensils and plastic wrap. Use a wooden hair brush with natural bristles.

Choose products that are packaged in glass instead of plastic containers. Store food in glass instead of plastic. Avoid synthetic fabrics—flooring, clothes, upholstery and linens. Lessen, as much as possible, your exposure to foam rubber, glues, inks, paints, varnishes, solvents, particleboard and plywood. Keep your car windows down as much as possible. Never burn garbage since it can release dioxin and PCBs into the air.

As we become more aware of the negative impacts of plastic and PVC on our individual health and the environment, reject plastic products and actively seek out other options in all aspects of your life. By introducing fewer chemicals into your life, you *will* become less toxic, a difficult goal, but not an impossible one.

UPHOLSTERY, TEXTILES, INKS & DYES

Harmful pollutants in textile manufacturing range from Volatile Organic Compounds (VOCs) to mineral solvents in print paste or inks. Harmful chemicals are also found in fire retardants and sealants used on fabric and upholstery. These substances can emit toxic

Telling you to avoid plastic would be like telling you to avoid breathing.

gases that cause illness. It is important to understand that the term organic, even with organic fabrics, refers to the growing methods of the material and not the way it is processed. Although much less than traditionally manufactured fabric, organic material sometimes contains chemicals, added in the finishing stages, which can give off gases. Most synthetic fabrics require more energy and chemicals than their natural equivalents during the manufacturing process.

Printing inks and dyes can be full of harmful chemicals, such as formaldehyde, acetone, hexavalent chromium and others. Permanent markers, clothing dyes and soy or natural-based dyes all come with the risk of contamination to the person manufacturing them. Toxic air emissions are a result of the manufacturing practices that produce dyes and inks.

Water-based and all natural dyes are safer choices; however, even these are not 100 percent environmentally and human friendly. Contact the EPA for guidelines and regulations. Color your world safe!

► **Consider** that some manufacturers are making the transition toward producing greener textiles by using organic dye extracts. Earth- and human-friendly fabrics and blends such as silk, hemp, cotton, wool, linen, ramie, papyrus, rubber, damask, and nettle are greener choices than their synthetic counterparts. Other natural fibers, such as sisal, coir and jute are used in coarse fabrics and floor mats.

WINDOW COVERINGS

Heavy cloth drapes can collect dust and mildew and usually require dry cleaning.

► **Consider** choosing natural fibers when selecting window coverings. Bamboo blinds and shades are a great choice because they are light, easy to clean and a sustainable resource that quickly grows back.

Office

ENVELOPES & LABELS

Stationery, stamps and other office products that use glue as a sealant contain chemicals that should not come in contact with your tongue.

► **Consider** using a sponge instead.

OFFICE MACHINES

Offices use huge amounts of energy, especially electricity, for heating, air conditioning, lighting, lifts and escalators, automatic doors, computers, printers, photocopiers, fax machines and much more. They use resources, generate waste, and can grow to be a toxic environment.

▶ **Consider** creating a green office. A green office is a smarter and better office. It is ecological in the sense that it uses nontoxic, recycled, environmentally-friendly products and supplies. Using as little energy and other resources as possible, a green office operates efficiently, thereby producing a smaller amount of waste. It provides a healthy work space with a minimum amount of visual noise and physical pollution. A green office uses energy-efficient lighting and office equipment, relying on natural light whenever possible. Everything is recycled from paper to printer cartridges; e-mail and telecommuting is strongly encouraged. The green office has nontoxic, durable, recyclable flooring, carpets, wall coverings, paints and furnishings.

Purchasing office machines that save energy will also prevent pollution. The Environmental Protection Agency (EPA) created the label Energy Star for products that meet strict energy-efficient criteria. The Energy Star label makes it easy for you to recognize the most efficient office machine models for computers, printers, scanners, fax machines and more. Over a lifetime, Energy Star qualified equipment in a home office including a computer, monitor, printer, and fax can save enough electricity to light an entire home for more than four years. Power managed machines, such as Energy Star use much less electricity than those without such power management features.

Copiers are the most energy-intensive type of office equipment because they sit idle for long periods of time. Powering down office machines when not in use for long periods of time can save energy, money and reduce pollution.

A green office is also a healthy office. Not only do employees feel better working there, but they may make fewer mistakes and get work done more efficiently. They also use fewer sick days. Many companies have already found that greening their offices has increased their employees' productivity so much that it has given them a competitive edge. Increases in productivity have helped many businesses pay for renovations even more quickly than they had anticipated. Studies have shown that when a workplace is made more energy-efficient and less toxic, increases in profits have been over ten times the norm from improved employee health and their heightened productivity.

When a workplace is made more energy-efficient and less toxic, increases in profits have been over ten times the norm.

Easy actions such as using a ceramic mug instead of throwaway cups or permanent, refillable tape dispensers instead of disposable ones will make a difference. Reusing envelopes and boxes by affixing a new label over an old one is another simple way to make a difference. Recycle, recycle and recycle office paper.

Using these considerations to create a green office can save money for a company, can benefit the environment by reducing pollution and the demand for resources and can make employees feel better physically and emotionally.

PAPER, PENS, PENCILS, INKS & DYES

Theoretically, the computer age was supposed to reduce our use of paper, but then again, home-videos were supposed to put cinemas out of business. Paper is the second largest consumer of chlorine after polyvinyl chloride (PVC) production. Chlorine that is used to whiten fibers from tree pulp produces dioxins that are a known carcinogen. Globally, trees are being cut at the rate of 75 acres per minute or 5,000 square miles a month. The average American uses and discards 700 pounds of paper per year, enough to build about a 12 foot wall from New York to Los Angeles!

According to the Natural Resources Defense Council, the virgin-timber based pulp and paper industry is the single largest industrial consumer of forests worldwide, the largest industrial consumer of freshwater and the largest generator of polluted wastewater. The industry is the third largest industrial generator of greenhouse gases and the fourth largest consumer of fossil fuels.

Just as in other mega-industries, big paper mills supply big printing companies who have an inordinate influence on politicians who vote in enormous subsidies to continue to support the problem, regardless of the cost to our Earth and your resources. Due to lower demand and developmental expenses, the cost to print on tree-free, sustainable fiber paper is usually more costly than heavily subsidized wood pulp which is neither sustainable nor recyclable. Currently their are few alternatives to printing on virgin-timber paper. The good news is that more post-consumer waste and fiber papers are being developed.

Recycled paper is a misunderstood phrase. Recycled paper, unless labeled as "post-consumer," is a byproduct of making paper with virgin-forested paper. Authentic *recycled* paper, labeled post-consumer waste, has been recovered from other uses, remade and recycled into usable paper. Other countries are leading the charge toward using sustainable fibers and authentically recycled papers as they see their timber resources evaporate.

▶ **Consider** that we all have to start doing what is right, not what is just cheap and convenient. Whenever possible, use recycled paper made from post-consumer materials. Recycled paper is not 100 percent green; however, it requires less chemicals than making paper from virgin wood.

When we make decisions based on doing what is right versus doing what is cheap or convenient, it will positively impact the toxic paper industry. Start by choosing post-consumer, recycled or sustainable fiber papers that are chlorine-free. When purchasing paper for your home or office, make an environmentally responsible decision. Choose alternative papers. This book is printed on New Leaf EcoBook paper that is 100% post consumer waste recycled, chlorine-, solvent- and heavy metal-free. New Leaf Paper is the industry leader in environmentally responsible and economically sound printing and office paper. The slightly higher cost for paper was worth it considering the trees and our resources that were saved. Thank you New Leaf.

Other sources for sustainable paper include fiber crops such as hemp and kenaf (kuh-naf). They require less chemicals and energy and can be processed in a chlorine-free environment. More trees are spared and the paper is produced with minimal impact to the environment. With additional demand from public interest and research funding, recycled and sustainable fiber paper has the potential to become a mainstream source for paper, preserving forest ecosystems. Other sustainable paper fibers being developed include, sugar cane stalks, cereal straw, corn husks and bamboo. (See Sources.)

Many printed materials, such as books, newspapers, phone books and magazines are printed and then stacked or wrapped in plastic which seals in the chemicals from the ink. If you are chemically sensitive, the papers may need to be opened and aired out before you read them. If possible, put them outside in the sunshine to dry and release some of the chemicals inherent in them.

Cut down on your paper habit by using e-mail. Although letter writing is a wonderful art, e-mail uses less energy to transport and sort. Even with the concerns about obsolete computers adding to our landfills, e-mail is still a more environmentally-friendly option to save on excess paper usage. In addition, just imagine the amount of wood, plastic, adhesives, and lead saved by not using stamps, pencils and pens.

Be creative and reuse paper products such as newspaper, gift bags, calendars, and maps. Your buying and recycling decisions will keep the pressure on the paper industry to produce more recycled paper products. This consumer demand has already led the paper

Keep using your recycling bin and do not believe any anti-recycling hype.

industry to invest in more and more recycling mills. Keep using your recycling bin and do not believe any anti-recycling hype.

If you prefer to do your bill paying by check, there are several recycled check companies available for both the individual and business. Often times, these companies also donate a percentage of the profit to positive environmental or social issues and endeavors. Remember that you can pay your bills online or perhaps with a credit card to reduce paper waste.

The U.S. population discards 1,600,000,000 pens per year. Colored pencils and non-toxic crayons are excellent alternatives to pens, permanent markers and toxic highlighters. Be a trendsetter; preside over your next meeting with a colored pencil in hand.

PUBLIC PLACES

Hospitals, schools, sporting arenas, retail stores, hotels, cruise ships, airplanes, institutions, restaurants and office buildings are typically built with toxic materials *and* cleaned with toxic chemicals. These chemicals can irritate the lungs and skin, causing rashes or aggravating asthma. Sick spaces result in sick people. Where do you put yourself in the course of the day? Are those spaces toxic? If so, protect yourself.

On some level, we are all somewhat familiar with the ancient art of Feng Shui— bringing the balance of nature into man-made environments. Compare the energy of a waterfall to a stagnant pond, fresh air to musty air, a state park to a strip mine and an organic farm to a landfill—the first environment will always feel better. When you walk into a space and immediately feel relaxed and secure, it is usually the result of balanced Feng Shui. On the contrary, spaces that evoke confusion, chaos and coldness usually are out of balance.

▶ **Consider** that removing yourself from toxic environments is sometimes the easiest solution available. When that is not possible, imagine a positive white light surrounding you like a bubble for protection. In polluted spaces, wear a personal air filter and air your clothes out when you arrive home. In noisy spaces, wear ear plugs. In dark places, carry a flashlight. In sad spaces, carry a picture of your loved ones or your favorite place in nature. In warm rooms, think cool thoughts. In closed spaces, open a window or door. You are getting the idea. Each small step is a way to put balance into your body while in public places. All of these suggestions will help protect you, but the bigger problem, the cause, still needs to be addressed. (See Building Materials, Health Care and Hotels)

Outdoor

COMPOSTING

It is interesting to note that before human intervention, all organic materials on earth were completely composted and recycled back into the earth. For some, composting may seem like an insurmountable idea, but just stop for a moment and ponder the benefits of such a small effort.

An average person generates about 1500 pounds of trash annually whereas the amount of trash from a person that composts is just 375 pounds. That means that every year each American discards 1175 pounds of organic garbage that can be composted. That is a tremendous difference and *you* can make such a difference yourself.

It is a beautiful thing to return organic matter to the earth.

▶ **Consider** that composting can be simple. Everyday items like vegetable scraps, eggshells, coffee grounds, unbleached paper towels, dried leaves and other organic materials can be composted.

Start with a composting buddy. There are many schools of thought and books dedicated to composting. Find a person in your local community who is successfully composting and ask them to share their knowledge.

Many types of compost-specific containers for both indoor and outdoor use are available or just a hole dug in the ground can suffice. It is a beautiful thing to return organic matter to the earth.

GARDENING

According to the National Gardening Association, more than 85 million households enjoy the benefits of gardening. Gardening promotes responsible stewardship of our land, and physical and emotional health. It can infuse beauty into our lives and into our communities.

There is no replacement for the taste of a summer tomato picked right from the vine. The pleasures and rewards of gardening remind us of the flow of nature. Even a small patio pot or a window herb garden can lift your spirits.

Problems in a garden arise when we rush to kill the bugs. Often the first thought is to use toxic chemicals that in the long run weaken the plant. Weakened plants are a sign that they are stressed or undernourished.

Rainwater and irrigation can transport pesticides and chemical fertilizers from our lawns and gardens into street drains and empty into neighborhood waterways. These detrimental contaminants pollute your region's streams, lakes and rivers and inevitably harm aquatic life, plants, animals and humans.

▶ **Consider** that while the environmental problems of the world may seem beyond our control, you can make a difference right in your own backyard. Good gardening strategies create healthy plants, many of which will suffer fewer pest problems. Learn how to use less harmful methods for managing insects, pests, weeds and diseases before reaching for chemical controls.

Instead of dousing your garden with chemicals, you could establish an organic, essential environment. Organic environments invite plants to thrive. Nourish any stressed plants with natural substances, or move them to another spot. Many garden pests can be removed with your hands, a strong blast of water from the hose and pruning shears.

Use botanical insecticides as they break down rapidly, usually within a few hours or perhaps days. Another plus is that they are not usually accumulated in the environment. Synthetic pesticides are toxic to living things and consist of a chemical mixture produced in a laboratory. (See Insects & Rodents.)

Have your soil tested to establish your fertilizer needs and what you can do to correct any deficiencies that may surface. Kits are available in most plant stores that test the soil's pH levels. Sometimes local colleges or universities offer acid/alkaline services for a small fee.

Visit a nursery or plant center to discuss your concerns or to develop a control measure that will remedy the pest, disease or weed that has so boldly and defiantly thrust itself into your personal Garden of Eden. Most plant problems can be traced to inappropriate and stressed growing conditions. A well adjusted native plant will thrive and will remain free of insects and diseases.

Just like the human body, plants respond much better to natural materials, such as natural fertilizers and composted materials. And just like humans, a little love and attention and a lot less toxins can go a long way toward producing a happy and healthy garden and gardener.

When it comes to organic gardening and organic food, I need to mention an inspiring, remarkable person named Alice Waters. She is a visionary, teacher, author, organic gardener and true friend to the environment. Her restaurant, Chez Panisse in Berkeley, California revolutionized the model for farm-to-table dining—organic ingredients that are grown locally. One of her more recent projects is the Edible Schoolyard, which has introduced organic gardening to middle schools, turning parking lots into schoolyard gardens. Thank you Alice for your dedication to promoting gastronomic and ecological literacy.

Organic gardening provides a connection to our Earth and to the cycle of life through the plants that we grow. Throughout their cycle of birth, growth, harvest, death, rest and rebirth, plants give us the best example of energy-efficient, sustainable living—everything is recycled and nothing is wasted.

GOLF COURSES

Golf courses are under extreme scrutiny by governmental and environmental groups on behalf of their chemical and water-intensive practices. In an effort to maintain a manicured appearance and competitive playing surfaces, tons of chemicals and often toxic-emitting equipment are required. Often this upkeep uses more pesticides, fertilizer and herbicides than farmland.

Now, I do not propose that people are going to play less golf because of this statement, but awareness leads to change. For those who are in the position to make decisions about how a course is maintained, make better choices based on the technologies that are more earth- and human-friendly.

▶ **Consider** that more and more courses are trying to improve their toxic chemical and water guzzling customs. Some golf courses are using recycled water and electric-powered equipment. When you are on the links, remember that the club and ball that you continually touch is coming in contact with many chemicals. Wash your hands as soon as possible.

If golf courses became "green" habitats, they could provide a much needed refuge for wildlife in suburban settings.

If golf courses became "green" habitats, they could provide a much needed refuge for wildlife in suburban settings. The United States Golf Association (USGA) and Audubon International have joined forces to create a program to promote ecologically sound land management and conservation on golf courses. Almost 2000 golf courses around the world have joined this program. For a list of participating courses that are fully certified, visit www.usga.org/green/environment/Audubon_program.html. If we could link creating essential environments with lowering golf handicaps, we might be on to something.

INSECT REPELLENT

Many insect repellents contain DEET (N.N-diethl-meta-toluamide or *N,N*-diethyl-3-methylbenzamide) which has been reported to have side affects ranging from rashes to seizures. Approximately 70 different companies use DEET in more than 200 different products. The EPA states that DEET is only "*slightly toxic.*" This reminds me of a saying used by authors William McDonough and Michael Braungart in their book *Cradle to Cradle*, "less bad is no good." Another chemical prevalent in insect repellent is permethrin, a suspected carcinogen and endocrine disruptor that can cause some people to have an acute allergic reaction.

For some reason insects love me. I have tried every safe alternative insect repellent on the market and have even resorted to making my own using essential oils. Those that worked were the ones containing citronella. I do not like the smell and neither do the bugs. The suggestion to tuck a dryer sheet on your hat keeps bugs away because they are repelled by the chemicals! This *is not* something you want to consider.

▶ **Consider** using insect repellents that do not contain DEET. Never use insect repellents on infants and read the label before applying them to young children. Sometimes the best protection and the least smelly is to cover your skin with clothing—long pants, long sleeved shirts and hats. Sweatshirts and pants made out of mosquito netting are available at most camping stores. These really do work. It also helps if you avoid being outside before dawn and after dusk when bugs are the most active.

Prevent ticks and tick-borne diseases through prevention. Avoid tick-infested areas. Stay on the path when hiking. Wear long pants and tuck them into boots. If insect repellent with DEET is your only option, spray it only on your clothes and avoid skin, eyes, mouth and face. Make sure to wash your hands after application.

Many nontoxic insect repellents are available. My favorite repellent does not contain citronella. It is an herbal spray by Garden's Alive!® that is called *Sting-Free Insect Bite Protector*. (See Sources.)

INSECTS & RODENTS

Grasp the idea that pesky bugs and rodents only come into your space when they know that they are going to find food. The non-pesky insects are labeled "beneficial insects" for their use as biological pest controls. Lady bugs, dragonflies, praying mantises, bats and damselflies eat many insects that pester plants and humans such as aphids and mosquitoes.

▶ **Consider** that the more organic your home and garden become, the less stressed your environment will be and you will attract fewer pests.

All pesticides are toxic. They do not know the difference between bugs and humans. Unfortunately, 90 percent of pesticides have never been tested for their effects on the human body. To control fleas, roaches, ants, etc., use diatomaceous earth, boric acid, and nematodes. Diatomaceous earth, a white-powdery substance made of pulverized sea shells, is odorless, stainless and can be used as pest control for small insects. These items are usually available at gardening stores, health food stores, and some pet supply stores.

Ever wonder how ants find there way back to the hill? They secrete invisible pheromone tracks so they and fellow ants can find their way back from foraging sites. Washing your floors and household surfaces with an equal portion of distilled white vinegar and water will remove this secretion and deter ants from returning. Then remove, seal or contain the food that attracted them in air tight containers or the refrigerator. Also, squirt apple cider vinegar along the outside foundation of your home or building to deter ants from entering. Barriers to control ants can be made by dusting borax where they enter.

There is always hope.

Another pest and insect deterrent is an ultrasonic device that you plug into a wall outlet. They use very little energy. The sound does not affect household pets or humans, but sends an ultrasonic wave through the walls encouraging insects and pests to move out of your space. Avoid plugging them into places where you spend a lot of time to reduce any exposure to electromagnetic fields that they may emit. (See Sources)

Bats are effective in controlling insects. Bats can eat up to 1,200 bugs such as mosquitoes and crop-destroying moths per hour. Bats are not dangerous vampires, they are our friends. Install a bat house on your property. Bats like their houses in sunlight, near water and at least 12 feet off the ground, preferably on a house where predators cannot get to them. Some organic farmers have had success using bat houses to attract bats to patrol orchards and consume insects.

Use humane pest control. It is not the animal's fault that they happen to cross your path. Visit your local home store or landscape nursery for other humane solutions.

LITTER

Chances are that if you are reading this book, you do not litter. A person that litters is terribly disconnected from the earth and her treasures. How unfortunate that our pathways and highways are filled with so much litter that we need to adopt lands to assure that they are cleared of litter.

▶ **Consider** that even a cigarette butt is litter. Until the consciousness level reaches a point that puts programs like Adopt-A-Highway out of business, adopt one! You can also start by adopting your business grounds, your backyard and your street. Enlist your co-workers, friends and family members to help. There is nothing more appealing than litter-free vistas. Non-litterers unite.

Billboards are best described as litter and visual clutter. In the past, Lady Bird Johnson supported the passage of legislation to ban billboards from our interstate highways. Due to the heavy opposition from advertising entities, the bill did not stick. Image how much more peaceful driving would be today if our vistas were of nature instead of steel, lights and pictures of beer bottles, cigarettes and cleavage!

There is always hope. The 17 mile stretch of pristine highway in Pennsylvania from Dunmore to Carbondale, called the Robert P. Casey Highway, has been designated a scenic highway to protect it from the pressure of outdoor media companies to erect billboards. Congratulations to these visionaries. Other drives such as Route 163 in California from Mission Valley to downtown San Diego remind us of how beautiful the vista can be without a billboard blocking the view.

YARDS

Reasons to grow and maintain grass might be to enjoy the feel of it under our feet, watch our children and pets play on it or to lie down on it on a hot day. Why else would we spend $25 billion annually growing 20 million acres of a crop that we can not eat, wear or sell? Unfortunately better lawns through chemicals do not support your health.

In addition to the toxic emissions of lawn equipment, over 70 million tons of fertilizers are applied to lawns each year. Lawn chemicals that are not organic are harmful to your children and pets, the birds and bees and all living things. That is why the chemical lawn companies place a sign in yards advising you not to sit on the grass for a period of time after they have sprayed chemicals.

▶ **Consider** on your small piece of the planet that you could reduce or eliminate unwanted chemicals and emissions to maintain a manicured lawn. Here are a few considerations that will help you maintain a chemical-free yard:

> ← *Check for organic gardeners' associations in your region to find to ways to improve your soil since healthy soil is important to maintaining a chemical-free*

lawn. Add earthworms, compost and manure to your yard to return natural nutrients to the soil. Use only organic fertilizers.

- Plant as much of your yard as possible in indigenous perennial plants and ground covers that take less resources to maintain.
- Cut grass at a higher level to reduce water usage and to shade weed seeds that will slow their growth. Let the clippings lay where they are cut.
- Avoid weed killers since they put yards under stress and can kill worms and beneficial insects. Avoid them. Keeping a lawn healthy naturally eliminates unwanted insects. Become one with the dandelions. If you must, dig them out the old-fashioned way.
- Select the proper grass for your area. I planted a short-growing blue fescue that does not need to be cut in my yard. It creates a wonderfully lush organic carpet.
- Have your community or neighborhood enact stricter regulations for using lawn-treatment chemicals because of the potential danger they pose to children and the population at large.

As mentioned before, authenticity is important in generating the flow of nature, especially in your yard. Authenticity comes from using plants that compliment a setting, not those that change it into something entirely different. If you live in a desert, plant desert landscaping, not water-hungry grass. Use indigenous plants to compliment your dwellings. Your backyard can become an environment that supports, not compromises your health.

Would you eat your bar of soap or drink your shampoo?

Personal Care

BATH & BEAUTY PRODUCTS

As the largest organ, the skin plays a critical role in eliminating toxins from your body. Would you eat your bar of soap or drink your shampoo? The regulations governing the use of the word organic in food production does not apply to personal care products. At present, the standards for the products that come in contact with our skin do not have the same safeguards as those that we ingest.

Manufacturers are using this consumer misunderstanding to exploit and capitalize on the increased demand for "organic" products. Surely you have noticed the shelves being flooded with "organic" bath and beauty products, most of which contain synthetic chemicals, such as sodium lauryl sulfate, olefin sulfonate, sodium myreth, fatty acids, methyl paraben, cocamidopropyl betaine and hundreds of other synthetics that are definitely inorganic. Any ingredient with "-eth" in its name are ethoxylated with ethylene oxide from petroleum and contain traces of dioxin, a highly toxic carcinogen. This battle over the chemicals used in organic personal care products is currently taking place between industry and government.

Your opinion matters. Contact the United States Department of Agriculture's (USDA) office of the National Organic Program to state your opinion on this subject- nop. webmaster@usda.gov, 202 720-3252. To keep tabs on this current event, visit www. organicconsumers.org/bodycare.

Support companies that are known for their human- and earth-friendly products and philosophy. The good news is that there are many companies devoted to your health and a sustainable environment. These companies are listed under Sources and include all personal care products from deodorants and shaving cream to shampoo and cosmetics. They are usually less expensive and more effective than conventional, chemical-laden products. The companies whose products are discussed have not exerted any influence on my opinion or content.

Now that you know that the word "organic" on personal care products is not regulated, protect your skin and become an ingredient-savvy customer. Manufacturers that list the products' ingredients on the label or their website usually do not have anything to hide. A great resource for understanding the ingredients on cosmetic and personal care products is *A Consumer's Dictionary of Cosmetic Ingredients* by Ruth Winter, M.S.

Contrary to what marketers would have you believe, antibacterial products have no impact on viruses. Overuse of antibacterial soaps may lead to underdeveloped immune systems and to super strength home bacteria, such as those that are already being fought by hospitals. Although antibacterial may sound like a good concept, it may actually cause more problems and weaken the bacteria your body uses to strengthen its immune system. An environment does not have to be sterile to be safe; in fact, a little less obsession with disinfecting everything may be better. Unless medically recommended, choose non-antibacterial products.

Fragrances and perfumes are a source of added chemicals in personal care products. You can read more about the caustic effects of fragrances in the Air Chapter. Select fragrance-free products to reduce your chemical intake and save the person next to you who may not like your selection of chemicals.

Band-aids. Here is another unsuspecting product that we may not recognize as toxic. Band-aids can contain latex which uses ammonia in its preserving process.

▶ **Consider** that if you are allergic to latex, sterile latex-free band-aids that do not use animal testing are available.

Body sponges & brushes. Body brushes or cloths made out of plastic are synthetic, not natural.

▶ **Consider** using natural bristle brushes made out of wood and palm plant fibers or boar bristle is a better choice for cleaning your skin. My favorite washcloth is made from the fiber of agave cactus by Ayate.

Cosmetics. As mentioned under labeling, cosmetic and beauty products do not have strict regulations governing their ingredients.

▶ **Consider** that safe, ecological make-up is available. My favorite companies are Aubrey Organics, Aveda, Burt's Bees, Ecco Bella and Dr. Hauschka. I trust these companies because their products are quality, safe, and ecological.

These companies also have an essential environment's mindset. For example, Aveda's mission is to "care for the world we live in, by the products we make to the ways in which we give back to society." They believe in conducting business in a manner that protects the earth, conserves resources and does not compromise the ability of future generations to sustain themselves. Good job, Aveda.

Deodorant. The health issues raised about aluminum chlorohydrate and other chemical compounds used in traditional deodorants and antiperspirants have caused a demand for alternative deodorants. When did we start to believe that our underarms are supposed to be dry? The pores under our arms and on the rest of our body are part of a pretty neat cooling system that removes the toxins from our body. Antiperspirants shrink the sweat glands thereby reducing perspiration and wetness. Deodorants also mask body odor with a chemical-laden scent.

▶ **Consider** that this is one place, close to your heart, where you can rid chemicals from your life. I use Thai Roll-on Deodorant which contains just salt and water.

When did we start to believe that our underarms are supposed to be dry?

Now, before you start worrying about your body odor, it works great and does not contain any harmful chemicals. You may need to adjust to your armpits becoming wet occasionally, but the trade-off is definitely worth it. Be aware that foods containing caffeine such as coffee, soft drinks and chocolate may accelerate body odor. What a great excuse to wean yourself off caffeine. Dusting your armpits with baking powder is another alternative for a safe, non-toxic deodorant.

Feminine hygiene products. The Toxic Shock Syndrome (TSS) scare associated with feminine hygiene products should remind us that any product we wear close to our bodies should be free and clear of toxins and fragrances. Keep in mind that traditional cotton is grown using as many as 35 different pesticides. Although industrial bleaching used in producing feminine hygiene products may contain only traces of dioxins, they are still dioxins, known as one of the most toxic chemicals ever produced.

▶ **Consider,** seriously consider, switching to 100 percent certified organic tampons—*today* if you have not already. Organic, biodegradable, non-chlorinated and perfume-free tampons, pads and panty liners are available.

For extremely chemically-sensitive women, other alternatives, such as organic Glad Rags can be used.

Hair care. Some shampoos are packed with alkaline chemicals and sudsing agents that can deplete essential oils from your hair. Other chemicals can build up on your hair leaving it dull and your scalp dry. Hair sprays can be very toxic in that they may contain butane, propane and nerve gas in an aerosol can.

▶ **Consider** healthy hair habits including eliminating or reducing the use of a hair dryer by letting your hair dry naturally, covering your hair when in the sun and wind, gently patting your hair to dry, and massage your scalp to improve circulation.

To help remove buildup from hair products, try a weekly rinse using organic apple cider vinegar. Mix 2 tablespoons of vinegar in a cup of water. Massage it into your hair after shampooing and leave it on for five minutes before rinsing.

Naturade's Aloe Vera 80 hair spray, made with aloe vera, is fragrance- and alcohol-free. Aubrey and Aveda have safe hair sprays in a pump spray. Also, plain aloe vera gel can be use as a hair gel.

Hair coloring & treatments. If letting your hair go gray naturally is not your preference, here is some good news. Reports show that the long-term use of traditional hair dyes does not cause cancer. They do, however, contain synthetic preservatives, coal tar dyes, phenylenediamine, resorcinol, ammonia and/or colors and synthetic fragrances. These harsh chemicals affect the environment and your skin.

Hair relaxers and permanent waves allow chemicals to enter your body through your scalp and skin. You should be suspect of any product that has a warning label.

▶ **Consider** using all-natural hair color. For years now, I have used natural hair color and love it. Not only does it produce great color, it does so without synthetic chemicals. It is gentle on my scalp and the condition of my hair is not compromised. The color is lasting and more natural. If you do not wish to experiment on your own, take it to your hair colorist and hopefully they too will consider converting to all-natural hair color!

New solutions are being created as the consumers' demand for earth- and human-friendly products increases. Currently, alternative solutions may not be available for treatments such as permanent waves and hair relaxers.

Hair removal. Men and women spend millions of dollars annually on products and services that promise hair removal. Over-the-counter hair removal products include shaving creams, waxes, tweezers, chemical depilatories and electrolysis tools. Many of these products are dispensed from aerosol cans and can contain chemicals such as lac-hydrin, ammonium lactate, ammonium hydroxide, calcium thioglycolate and glyceryl stearate.

▶ **Consider** that the type of hair removal you choose to protect your skin depends on the amount of hair growth and the area to be treated, as well as the safety, effectiveness, cost and type of method. A professional salon can advise you on the methods and their associated costs.

The most cost-effective, natural methods for hair removal are shaving with non-toxic products, tweezing and waxing. Read the labels on hair removal products and select those that are safe and nontoxic such as Kiss My Face shaving cream, Aubrey's Herbal Mint/Ginseng shaving cream and Burt's Bees shaving soap. If your skin is extremely sensitive, 100 percent aloe vera gel that is available at health food stores can be used instead of shaving cream. Avoid all products in aerosol cans.

> *New solutions are being created as the consumers' demand for earth- and human-friendly products increases.*

Lotions & sunscreens. With thousands of brands on the market, choosing a safe, moisturizing skin lotion or sunscreen can be time consuming, confusing and expensive. Even when your selection has been made, the product does not always produce the results you expected.

▶ **Consider** fragrance-free moisturizers that support and protect your skin. A company that deserves special mention is Aubrey Organics. For over 33 years, they have been the leader in natural hair and skin care products that are free of synthetics and petrochemicals. Their products are good both for the body and the earth. With over 140 hair, skin and body care products, they guarantee 100 percent natural and no animal testing. Furthermore, they have an essential environments mindset in that they have had their manufacturing facility certified organic. Now they are having all of their ingredients, hundreds of them, organically certified as well. Aubrey's Ultimate Moist and Sun Shade Ultra 15 are my favorite lotions.

For the chemically sensitive, plain olive, almond or coconut oil and cocoa butter are wonderful alternative lotions.

Body lotions are subjective and a personal choice, but at least now the selection has been simplified.

Nail polish. The nasty chemical in most nail polish is formaldehyde, followed by other nasty chemicals in nail polish remover and acrylic nail products. If you want to reduce the chemicals in your life, this is a good place to start.

▶ **Consider** letting your nails go natural. I wore fake nails for years in the 80s and had some anxiety about removing them. But to my surprise, it is one of the best things I could have done to become healthier and more authentic. It removed the nasty chemicals and, because of my restored health through making better food choices, my nails are strong and natural looking. I now use a natural nail system sold at beauty supply stores that buffs the nail and leaves a natural shine.

Personal care paper products. Chlorine bleach, perfumes and other chemicals can be present in paper products such as facial tissues, toilet paper, feminine hygiene products, and disposable diapers.

▶ **Consider** choosing fragrance- and chlorine-free products that are more earth- and human-friendly. Seventh Generation offers a wide selection.

Shoe polish. Many shoe polishes contain aerosol propellants or toxic solvents such as methylene chloride, nitrobenzene, perchloroethylene, trichloroethane, trichloro-ethylene, and xylene.

► **Consider** that a combination of 2 teaspoons of olive oil with a few drops of lemon juice can be applied with a thick cotton or terry cloth rag for an all natural shoe polish. Leave it on for a few minutes; wipe and buff with a clean, dry rag. Beeswax can also be used in a formula with olive oil and earth pigment. For this and other formulas for making your own non-toxic household cleaning products refer to Annie Berthold-Bond's *Better Basics for the Home.*

Skin care. Frustration with so many personal care products is that they offer promises that do not materialize. Again, simplifying is the key and this information will help you to minimize your choices and maximize your results.

► **Consider** using products from these companies that offer great skin care lines that are non-toxic and beneficial to your skin: Aubrey Organics, Dr. Hauschka, Aveda, Burt's Bees and Zia Natural Skin Care.

For those not familiar with Dr. Hauschka, it is a skin care company which has been practicing biodynamic cultivation of medicinal plants since 1935. In addition to providing a great skin care line, they are experienced in the use of natural substances and the conservation of nature. Hauschka's quality control of skin care products follows pharmacopoeia guidelines.

For the chemically sensitive, use cocoa butter, plain olive or almond oil.

Soap. Not all soaps are created equal. Many have harsh chemicals that deplete the natural oils from your skin and add toxicity to your life. Just like other body care products and detergents, avoid soaps that contain harmful chemicals such as sodium lauryl sulfate, phosphate salts and other synthetic ingredients listed above.

► **Consider** using an unscented, pure olive oil or coconut oil soap. Look for natural ingredients in soap such as vegetable-oil based, almond, vitamin E and apricot oil.

Although there are many safe soap and body care manufacturers, I want to especially mention Burt's Bees. They have built an empire on the foundation of natural body care. Their products do not contain petroleum-synthesized fillers or artificial preservatives that may irritate the skin. Water-based products include such ingredients as beeswax, plant oils and natural colors. Of course, their packaging is recyclable. I love their peppermint shower soap. Dr. Bronner's liquid castile, vegetable-oil soaps are also good alternatives.

Toothpaste. The proliferation of over 500 brands of specialty toothpastes has caused much confusion as to which is the best choice. The two controversial ingredients in toothpaste are saccharin and fluoride. Saccharin, a synthetic sweetener 400 times sweeter than sugar and a possible carcinogen, is used in most major brand name toothpastes on the market today. Fluoride is toxic in its pure form, but the amount in toothpaste, if used properly, will keep fluoride ingestion to a minimum. The controversy over fluoride is discussed in the Water Chapter and relates mostly to mass fluoridation of municipal drinking water.

▶ **Consider** Tom's of Maine, Jason, Nature's Gate, and Kiss My Face, a few of the companies that offer selections that are safe and non-toxic. For the chemically sensitive, baking powder works great. Whatever your toothpaste preference, gel, paste, or even powder, choose one that does not add chemicals to your life.

CELEBRATIONS

Sometimes it is difficult to realize that our culture's traditional celebrations can harm the earth. Seemingly innocent decorations such as festive balloons which are released into the atmosphere deflate and land in areas where animals can get tangled in the string or even die from ingesting them. In addition, they are not biodegradable.

Fireworks pollute the air and plastic party favors consume more of our resources.

The ink used on most gift wrap is not biodegradable, yet Americans spend $2.9 billion a year on wrapping paper, ribbons and gift bags. Tons of paper products and single-use plastic ware that quickly becomes trash is a by-product of our celebrations. The information on wrapping paper alone motivated me to find ways to create healthier, more responsible celebrations.

▶ **Consider** that celebrations can be an occasion to create essential environments with earth- and human-friendly items. Decorate with recycled paper, make balloon shapes or create festive mobiles. Give non-toxic personal care products, safe candles, organic herbal teas or essential oils as party favors. Bake a cake using organic ingredients and use beeswax birthday candles. Celebrate in ways that conserve our resources and your health. Make each celebration you have a celebration of the earth and all it has to offer us by not harming ourselves and our environment.

Solutions to environmentally friendly gift wrap are easy. One can readily make a gift look exciting in an essential way. There is always the old standby of using old maps, magazines or brown paper bags decorated with non-toxic paints and markers. The Asian culture uses scarves as gift wrap. Since this could become a bit costly, in its place you can use natural fiber fabric remnants, such as cotton, linen or silk for wrapping your presents. Use any scrap fabric lying around or visit a fabric store for remnants. Lay the present on the piece of fabric, take two opposite corners and tie them in a knot. Then take the two remaining corners and make a knot on top of the first knot. This makes a festive, reusable and recyclable gift wrap. At the very least, try using gift bags that can be reused.

Although paper products are convenient for party cleanup, a few dishes among friends are a better solution.

Although paper products are convenient for party cleanup, a few dishes among friends are a better solution than sending these products to a landfill where they may sit for the next 200 years or more. Instead of plastic ware, use your everyday utensils. For large family gatherings, restaurant supply stores sell inexpensive stainless utensils and other eco-friendly options. If you must use paper, buy post-consumer, recycled versus styrofoam. Post-consumer means that a product uses previously-used paper versus using the waste from virgin-forested paper.

Do without beverages in plastic bottles. Instead, serve juice or iced tea in pitchers or spring water in glass bottles. Serve beverages in glass or paper cups that can be reused or recycled.

Opt for dish towels instead of paper towels as they can be laundered and reused. If paper towels are the only option, buy those that are unbleached, recycled, and dioxin-free.

CLOTHING

Clothes made with synthetic fibers such as polyester, Lycra, rayon, spandex, Gore-Tex, vinyl and Tencel are prepared using petroleum. Your body can absorb unnecessary chemicals when these fibers lay against your skin. Permanent press and wrinkle resistant clothes have been treated with formaldehyde, a chemical that does not wash out of clothing. A few wrinkles seem much less threatening than the contaminants that prevent them.

Traditional cotton T-shirts are usually printed with synthetic dyes, harmful solvents and PVC plastic. This process can use up to one-third pound of chemicals per shirt. If that is not bad enough, traditional methods of growing cotton employ pesticides, herbicides and synthetic fertilizers.

▶ **Consider** wearing clothes that are made with natural, organic fibers—100 percent cotton, silk, linen, hemp or wool. These sustainable sources do not contain petroleum. This may be a bigger challenge than you want to embrace, but a wider selection of stylish organic clothing is becoming available. Use organic and natural fibers when selecting baby clothes.

As awakening continues, companies such as Nike and IKEA have phased-out the use of toxic PVC in their products.

Manufacturers of organic clothing and other organic products pledge that pesticides, harsh resins, plastics and sweatshop labors *are not* used.

If permanent press clothes are your only option, soak them in powdered milk and then launder to remove most of the formaldehyde before wearing them. This process will help to leach out the chemicals that are in the fiber. At the very least, wear T-shirts, socks and undergarments that are crafted from natural fibers since they come in direct contact with your skin.

Instead of using mothballs when storing clothes, use cedar chips or sachets filled with herbs such as rosemary, mint or lavender.

For the truly dedicated, hide-free, compostable shoes made out of hemp and natural fiber sewing notions are available. (See Sources.)

DENTAL HYGIENE

Good dental hygiene is required to create and sustain an essential environment in your mouth. Regarding the safety of materials and practices related to dental health, we are once again faced with differences of opinion.

Amalgam or silver colored fillings are 50 percent mercury plus other metals including silver, copper, zinc and tin. High levels of mercury exposure can cause permanent damage to the brain, kidneys and developing fetuses. The debate over the amount of mercury exposure received from these fillings and our threshold to its harmful effects continues without a general consensus. Reputable scientific studies have failed to find any link between amalgam restorations and any medical disorder. Regardless of these findings, mercury is a toxin; and if you are concerned about or sensitive to this, choose an alternative substance. Talk to your dentist about your concerns; he or she will assist you in your decision to avoid any toxic material in your dental care regimen.

Additional fillings include glass ionomers, resin ionomers and some composite (resin) fillings. These alternatives are a mixture of acrylic resin, acrylic acid and finely ground glass-like particles that make a tooth-colored material. Fillings, as well as other dental procedures, can include chemicals. Once again, make certain to discuss all of your options with your doctor. When in doubt, get a second opinion.

The practice of adding fluoride to drinking water is another issue that is far from being resolved. Studies have been conducted on both sides of the debate as to the effectiveness of fluoride which is added to thousands of water systems. Controversy exists over questions, such as does it actually protect against the loss of teeth into old age, is it safe to drink and does it increase the risk of oral cancer? Currently fluoridation levels are within the range recommended by the EPA. These fluoride levels were originally based on average water consumption alone. However, these levels have been thrown out of skew by additional fluoridated water consumption in processed food and drink such as baby food, juice and soft drinks.

My family has been in dentistry for the last 60 years and in their collective experience they have seen thousands of children—some who have had fluoridated water or low levels of fluoride from toothpaste and some who have not. They told me the difference is staggering. Those who had fluoride had significantly better oral health. Now that you have heard both sides, you can judge for yourself.

If you are concerned about your fluoride intake, use a water filter designed to remove fluoride. There are some scientists calling for an end to the practice of fluoridation. The verdict is still out but you can arrive at an informed decision.

Oral products that you use daily to clean your teeth are most likely full of chemicals. Chances are the mint or cinnamon flavor in your dental floss is made of chemicals. The wax on dental floss and mouth wash could add more chemicals to your dental hygiene routine.

▶ **Consider** that, in general, dentists and other medical practitioners need to continue to discuss and investigate ways to keep their patients as well as their offices environmentally safe.

Replace your chemical-laden floss, toothpaste and mouthwash with products that are free of chemicals. Make sure that any flavoring is derived from an essential oil and not a synthetic additive. There are several brands and varieties available to satisfy your per-

Replace your chemical-laden floss, toothpaste and mouthwash with products that are free of chemicals.

sonal preference. Nature's Gate Cool Mint Gel and Jason's Power Smile are my favorite toothpastes. Tom's of Maine also offers a wide selection of safe, non-toxic toothpastes. (See Toothpaste under Personal Care Products in the Earth chapter.)

Most traditional style toothbrushes are made of nylon—another unnatural man-made product. Natural, sustainable products such as natural bristles and wooden handled toothbrushes are wonderful and great alternatives. I love the way the natural bristles feel when brushing my teeth and when it wears out I can put it in my compost pile or simply bury it in the ground to recycle. The next best thing to natural bristle toothbrushes are replaceable snap-on head toothbrushes. It is the head that wears out, not the handle. They are economical and ecological.

DRY CLEANING
Many dry cleaners have opted to stop using percoethylene, a chlorinated petroleum solvent that is widely used in the dry cleaning process. Check to see if your dry cleaner is among them. High levels of repeated exposure to this chemical can cause liver cancer in mice and memory loss in humans.

New products are being introduced to dry clean clothes and fabrics in home dryers. The process uses chemical and fragrance cloths in a dryer bag to clean clothes. Companies promoting these products would not reveal the ingredients leading us to deduct that the chemicals are not earth- or human-friendly.

▶ **Consider**, when possible, that the first line of defense for "dry clean only" clothes is to hang them outside to freshen. An option for removing odors from clothing is to put the item in the dryer on air fluff using a towel sprinkled with several drops of lavender essential oil. Many clothes that say "dry clean only" can be hand washed; only make sure you know what you are doing first. Buy clothes that do not need to be dry cleaned. When dry cleaning is absolutely necessary, make sure to remove the plastic bags immediately to air out the clothes or ask the dry cleaner not to bag them in the first place. Locate a "green" dry cleaner. Wearing natural fiber, chemical-free clothing against your skin helps to reduce your exposure to unwanted chemicals.

EYEWEAR
The development of contact lenses was a milestone in ophthalmic care. It solved many eye problems that previously could not be corrected with glasses. As with most innova-

tive developments, there is always a price to pay. Earlier versions proved to be toxic and required more care and hygiene. Newer lenses are made of materials that are *less* toxic and require less care.

▶ **Consider** that it is imperative to follow the directions for the care of the eyewear you choose. This will help to prevent adverse reactions and infections. If you are chemically sensitive, glasses are a better choice for keeping chemicals out of your eyes.

GIFT GIVING

Who needs another knick-knack?

I realized a few years ago that my personal gift giving had risen to an all time high. Just like food, material goods are cleverly marketed and have become less expensive and convenient to purchase, down to the perfectly-scripted greeting card. For me, the act of gift giving had lost its connection to the flow of nature; it did not resonate with my absolute choice of simplifying my life. So I decided to make a few changes. The biggest change appeared when I shared my feelings concerning my desire to create essential environments with my friends and family. Fortunately, they concurred and we changed our ritual of gift giving. It may sound as if I am using Grinch philosophy when actually my intention is to be more like the residents of Whoville. The gift of yourself and your time is a memorable and priceless one!

▶ **Consider** that you could evaluate your gift-giving practices. The most wonderful thing was that my friends and family were actually relieved by the unnecessary and often obligatory consumption associated with gift giving. Furthermore, it does not have any connection to how much we care for each other. In fact, honoring and respecting each other is the ultimate gesture of sincere and genuine caring. Perhaps when a person begins to become aware of the interrelatedness of the earth and ourselves, there is a natural spilling over of respect and concern for our fellow human beings.

We did agree, however, to give living gifts—gifts that support our health and the earth—the gift of listening, a home cooked meal, a plant instead of cut flowers, a recycled book, a homemade card or the gift of time, love and friendship. Give gifts that do not produce waste, such as concert tickets, gym memberships, charitable donations or museum passes. After all, who needs another knick-knack?

HEALTH CARE

This is another one of those complex topics that affects all of our lives—hospitals, doctor's offices, rehab centers, long-term care facilities, and waiting rooms. Do not even bother to stop and think about how environmentally-friendly your local hospital is because without question, it is not! PVC, pesticides, toxic cleaning solvents, chlorine, dioxins and waste are present in the majority of medical environments.

▶ **Consider** that there *is* hope. Health Care Without Harm is an international coalition of hospitals and health care systems, medical professionals, community groups, labor unions, environmental and religious organizations. This group is working to transform the health care industry into a sustainable mindset, one that is no longer a source of harm to public health and the environment. I know it sounds like a great idea, but it is an overwhelming task. Until this task is completed, be patient instead of being a patient!

What can you do to reduce the toxicity in health care? I advise you to save yourself first, but often times you have to position others on the path to help you. We all have to make the path. Asking questions about the medical products and practices employed is a good way to enlighten others that the current solution is not safe.

Until these spaces become clean and green, protect yourself when you are subjected to these environments. Studies prove that patients who have a view of nature heal faster and stay healthier longer—even if it is a picture and not the real thing. Tack a landscape picture or poster on your hospital wall. Use a personal air purifier when visiting a hospital or doctor's office. Take your own cotton sleep attire, non-toxic personal care products and stainless steel drinking mug. Bring your own water in glass bottles or use a water filter pitcher.

These suggestions may be small gestures at reducing your exposure to toxic pollutants in hospitals, but they are a start.

To further prevent the need for health care, continue removing and keeping the toxins out of our bodies. Personally, I prefer cooperative, healing modalities such as reflexology, acupuncture, massage, healing touch and aromatherapy. We take better preventative care of our automobiles than we do of our bodies. Cooperative healing modalities are a wonderful way to increase your resistance and prevent the toxins in your world from giving you a "breakdown."

INFANTS, CHILDREN & SCHOOLS

Unfortunately, our children are raised in homes and institutions that are not environmentally safe. The effects of harmful chemical exposure to our children and their resulting dis-eases are becoming more and more acknowledged. School buildings face significant problems including the possible existence of radon, lead, asbestos, outdated plumbing, sewage, termites, ventilation, dust, mold, chemical cleaners, germs and more.

The National School Lunch Program that serves approximately 29 million children daily is a disgrace. As a market for surplus high-fat and chemically-laden agricultural commodities, particularly beef and dairy products, the lunch program is in dire need of reform. Lunches offering pizza, hamburgers, hot dogs, nachos and sugary snacks have created three major food groups for children—fat, salt and sugar.

Another area of great concern to parents wanting to protect their children and their earth is disposable diapers. Ninety percent of American parents use disposable diapers on their babies, a plastic non-breathable material that may contain toxins that can be absorbed into a baby's skin and into our earth.

Over 18 billion diapers are thrown away annually. They comprise almost 12 percent of the trash that ends up in landfills. *Natural Home* Magazine states that one disposable diaper can outlive your children's great-great grandchildren. The diapers' toxic human feces can leach into groundwater contributing to viral illnesses. The dispute over cloth versus disposable diapers continues to be fueled from both sides of the landfill.

When you take into consideration all of the aspects related to diapers, from consumption of raw materials, waste, sewage, energy usage, air pollution and energy, neither type of diapering shows significant advantages. If using cloth diapers is overwhelming, you may want to use them in addition to disposable diapers.

The area of child care, including both infants and children, has made great advances and has created enormous conveniences. Alas, some of them have not been so friendly to our children or their environments. In her book *Having Faith*, which explores the ecology of pregnancy, Dr. Sandra Steingraber stresses the importance of an infant's first environment, a mother's womb. Using the solutions in these chapters will help you to create essential environments for your infants and children who are more susceptible to our chemical-laden wombs and world.

▶ **Consider** improving and protecting your child's environment. Simple steps can be taken to reduce and eliminate harmful chemicals and practices. Long-standing visionary and

Lunches offering pizza, hamburgers, hot dogs, nachos and sugary snacks have created three major food groups for children—fat, salt and sugar.

New York Times best-selling author, Doris J. Rapp, M.D., offers step-by-step help in detecting environmental illness in your child with an explanation of symptoms and diseases in *Is This Your Child's World?* (See Sources.)

Congratulations to Kelly Preston and Olivia Newton John who have become the spokeswomen for the movement committed to helping parents build healthy environments. Kelly is on the board of directors of the Children's Health Environmental Coalition (CHEC), a nonprofit organization that educates parents about protecting children from hazardous materials.

Children are born with a desire to eat organic food that is free of chemicals. As processed foods are introduced into their diet, they gradually stop listening to this desire. Providing pleasurable, nutritious whole foods that support your child's health is the best gift you can give them.

Ultimately, parents want to use the most natural products that would protect their children and their environment. If organic, cloth diapers, washed in free and clear detergent is not an option for you then use a wonderful alternative from Seventh Generation. They have researched and developed one of the most user- and eco-friendly disposable diaper on the market—free of dyes, fragrances, Tributyl tin (TBT), and chlorine. Other safe disposable diaper options include TenderCare Diapers and Tushies. These disposable diaper options may be better for your baby and easier to biodegrade, but they still end up in the landfill. While some solutions appear to be promising, they are only the first step toward more sustainable options. The next frontier will be eco-friendly diaper pails!

LABELING

In today's market, many products such as cleaning, bath and beauty products are not required to label their ingredient content. When contacting companies to request a list of ingredients used in their products, we were met with great resistance. The general mindset was that knowing what we were ingesting or exposing to our skin was not any of our business! One company required that a doctor request the list of chemicals. We had a doctor submit the request and found that many of the chemicals in their products were, indeed, toxic.

We also found the manufacturers that list their products' ingredients on the labels or their website usually do not have anything to hide. On the other hand, those that were vague or resisted the sharing of this information usually had some chemical to hide.

The bottom line of chemical use in products is that most of them have never been tested for their effects on the human body but several are known to cause ill health.

Manufacturers use words to make you think a product is safe, such as floral, natural, and hypo-allergenic. The word "unscented" on a label usually means that a chemical has been used to *mask* the smell of other ingredients. Choose fragrance-free labels. Hypo-allergenic products may contain other allergens, but usually not perfume.

When a product label announces *new and improved,* sometimes it is because some new chemical has been added, usually under the guise of bringing the consumer a better product, but not necessarily a safer or healthier one. In reality, the manufacturer probably instituted a new way to prolong shelf life or an improved way to increase productivity. Rarely is the supposed innovation more user- or earth-friendly. Be careful of *new and improved* products unless you really know what is in the product or what has been added or subtracted.

▶ **Consider** reading about the current struggle to keep integrity in organic labeling for non-food products under Personal Care, Bath & Beauty Products. Someday, hopefully soon, companies will be required by law to list *all* of the product's chemical ingredients, organic and non-organic, on the label. Until then, ask questions and refuse to buy products when the chemical content is not labeled or made available. For now, labels that say "organic" do not always mean they are good for you.

You are smart. Read labels and choose available alternatives that reduce the chemicals in your space and the toxins in your food. Look the four R's on labels—recyclable, refillable, reusable and/or returnable. Other words used on eco-friendly products are chemical-free, fragrance-free, biodegradable, free and clear, cruelty-free, latex-free, no animal testing and from sustainable resources.

A great resource for understanding the ingredients on cosmetic and personal care products is *A Consumer's Dictionary of Cosmetic Ingredients* by Ruth Winter, M.S.

PLANTS

There are many studies that show the benefits of plants in creating healthy spaces that enable occupants to have less stress and more focus. Some of the best household plants for removing toxicity and keeping your environments healthy are philodendrons, aloe vera, English ivy, golden pothos and Boston ferns. Vigorously healthy plants support an essential environment. Plants are soothing to our sight with their mysterious

You are smart. Read labels and choose available alternatives that reduce the chemicals in your space and the toxins in your food.

beauty and are pleasing to our disposition while they also supply extra oxygen as a fringe benefit.

When visiting an office environment, I can usually count on finding one or more struggling plants. You have seen these plants; they are in every office—the ones with tiny stems and a few leaves that are trying to survive. They look sad, spindly, and desperate for attention in the form of nourishment.

▶ **Consider** helping your office mates to let go of these plants that serve as a metaphor for struggle in your life. These plants are yearning to be returned to the earth—returned to the cycle of life. If possible, plant them outside of the building where adequate sunlight and moisture are readily available.

A few healthy houseplants can support better health. Place them near the area where you sit. Use a mild solution of soap and water to keep the leaves clean. Avoid leaf sprays as they contain chemicals. If actual plants are not feasible, use pictures of plants and trees to bring this healing energy into your space. At least you will not have to water them!

SHOES OFF, PLEASE

Much of the dirt and contaminants that enter your home are carried in on the bottom of shoes. When you retrace the steps your shoes have taken in a day, from public restrooms to parking lots, you will see how this is probable. Contaminants on the bottom of shoes such as lead, fuel, bacteria and pesticides are tracked onto your carpets and flooring where children play and pets roam.

▶ **Consider** that an easy solution is to remove your shoes at your front door. Your family and friends will enjoy revitalizing this old custom and you will enjoy a cleaner floor.

When repair people visit my home and need to wear their boots for protection, I give them boot covers made out of old blue jeans and elastic, similar to the shoe covers used in hospitals, only these are washable. They serve their purpose and are also machine washable, not disposable. Initially, people roll their eyes but then always ask where they can get a pair. Washable shoe covers can be found at hospital supply stores.

SUSTAINABLE INVESTING

Another way that an individual can make a difference in his or her social and physical environment is to integrate personal and social issues with investment decisions. The premise is similar to voting or to making your voice heard through your consumer choices. Tax dollars are very difficult to control and often offer little support to the larger issues that confront our society.

Investment dollars carry more of a clout because they can be used to support companies that are socially responsible. Out of this ability to endorse and influence with capital, the Pax World Fund was established. Instead of passively boycotting certain stocks, Socially Responsible Investing (SRI) is aimed at the opportunity to transform corporate policy for ethical reasons as opposed to mere financial gain.

In order to discover what stocks were "sin" stocks, those related to tobacco, alcohol, gambling or defense, responsible investors began to screen the companies to locate those with favorable social characteristics. Through such progress and foresight, we now have program-related investments that are both environmentally and financially successful.

Although you may not have that bronze glow, you could look smarter and be eco-chic going tan-less.

▶ **Consider** that you can assist in creating and maintaining superior companies, which are socially and environmentally sound, by investing intelligently and profiting consciously. Become a proactive investor who monitors the behavior of firms in your portfolio. You can reap positive returns by transferring the shareholders' concerns and impact from the living room to the board room. Today, there are over 144 socially responsible mutual funds available and SRI is establishing itself as a convincing presence in the investment community. For more information on such investments, visit the Pax website, www.pax.com. The rewards of a socially and ethically designed investment strategy feel good and benefit your essential environment. Put your money where your health and your heart are!

TANNING SALONS, LOTIONS & PILLS

On the average, 1 million Americans visit tanning salons each day. While you might feel better with an artificial tan, wearing the color of your natural skin is more authentic and could prevent more chemicals and dis-ease from entering your life. Ultra-violet rays from indoor tanning booths can be just as harmful as the sun's rays. One State is pushing Legislature to prevent children under 18 from using tanning salons.

Some salon sprays and many of the over-the-counter self-tanning lotions contain dihydroxacetone (DHA), dyes, tyrosine, preservatives and/or psoralens. Although advertising promotes UV-free and sunless tanning, the coloring agents that interact with the skin to darken it have not been tested for long-term effects. DHA tans give a false sense of protection from natural sun rays, when in fact they offer little protection.

Pills for self-tanning have not been approved by the FDA. They can contain canthaxanthin which has been approved in very small amounts as a food coloring additive. Ingesting enough of this chemical to tan your skin could cause serious health problems from liver damage to eyesight disorders.

Another reason to be cautious of the sun's rays is photosensitivity. Chemicals in many substances such as food additives, medications, deodorants, nylon and wool fibers, artificial sweeteners, antibacterial soaps, petroleum products, hair dyes, hair styling products, shoe polish and mothballs are considered photosensitizers. When exposed to UV radiation from natural or artificial sources, these photosensitizers can cause some individuals to become sensitive to light, resulting in a wide variety of health issues.

▶ **Consider** that although you may not have that bronze glow, you could look smarter and be eco-chic going tan-less. Our skin is a barrier for protecting the body from elements such as chemicals and sunlight, yet it is breathable and has its limits.

Using responsible actions, the sun can be our friend. Most doctors set the limit on 15 to 20 minutes of "natural sun" per day without sun block, depending on your skin type. This is usually enough to supply the required amount of vitamin D to decrease the risk of cancer, diabetes and other diseases. For those on medications or using any products containing photosensitizers, use sun precautions to prevent photosensitivity. Quite simply, over exposure to UV radiation from natural or artificial sources increases your risk of cancer.

Consult your doctor for clinical uses of self-tanning lotions for vitiligo (loss of skin pigmentation), spider veins or to shield individuals with photosensitivity disorders.

Pet Care

PETS

Scientists agree that animals can improve our psychological as well as our physical health. Whether you share a space with a bird, a dog, a turtle or a cat, they also need an essential living space. Pet food and paraphernalia, such as toys, beds, and blankets can be sources of toxicity so make your selections wisely. Sadly, more and more pets are becoming overweight and unhealthy due to a diet of non essential pet foods.

Each year pets are accosted with an array of toxic chemicals applied by their owners to kill fleas and ticks. Most sprays, dusts, flea collars and chemical dips are toxic to you and your pet. Unknowingly, many veterinarians use these toxic pet products on their furry and feathered patients. Not enough government testing of pet products and their impact in the home has been conducted. Many pet products on your grocery and pet store shelves contain pesticides and may be the reason for thousands of pets being killed through their exposure and application. The effects of toxic pet products can be a more worrisome scenario when young children and pregnant women are exposed to them.

Pet enthusiasts can even train their dogs and cats to use the toilet with an inexpensive seat attachment sold at most pet stores!

▶ **Consider** reading the labels when purchasing pet products and avoid commonly used harmful chemicals, such as chlorpyrifos, dichlorvos, phosmet, naled, tetachlorvinphos, diasinon, Malathion, carbaryl and propozur.

Read the label on pet foods and treats that you feed to your pet. Look for pet foods that do not contain chemicals, meat by-products, added colorings, flavorings or preservatives. PetGuard, Wysong and Blue Buffalo are my choices for pet food. Check company websites for a list of their products' ingredients. All the ingredients will not be organic; however, try to buy products that have the most real food ingredients.

If fleas and ticks are a problem, put fresh garlic or brewer's yeast in your pet's food. Freshen your pet's sleeping area with packets or dried herbs like rosemary, lavender or eucalyptus seeds wrapped in cheesecloth. Another alternative, Orange Guard, a natural pesticide derived from d-limonene (orange peel extract), is excellent for fighting fleas, ants and other small insects. It is water-based and can be used around food, both indoors and out.

Other safe practices to reduce the chemicals and fleas in you and your pet's life are to vacuum frequently and regularly comb your pet with a flea comb as you look for fleas. In more severe cases, or when a pet is allergic to fleas and needs immediate relief, use "insect growth regulators" or IGRs. Make sure the product manufacturer does not combine them with organophosphates, chlorpyrifos, dichlorvos, phosmet, naled, tetachlorvinphos, diasinon, Malathion. Two new pesticide products on the market are fipronil (marketed as Frontline or Topspot) or imidacloprid (marketed as Advantage).

Make sure pet toys are natural and that they are not chewing on plastic, PVC-based products that could leach chemicals into their systems. Select natural fiber materials in pet bedding. To keep added chemicals out of their lives and yours, use free and clear shampoo and detergents when bathing them or laundering their bedding.

PET LITTER

It has been reported that the perfume in cat litter can cause asthma. This is not surprising as most litter contains chemicals including phosphates.

Toxoplasmosis is a disease caused by a parasite that can be contracted through contact with cat feces, infected soil, litter boxes or undercooked meats or foods contaminated with the parasite. Pregnant women should avoid litter boxes, as these parasites can cross the placenta and cause severe birth defects or miscarriage. Have someone else volunteer to clean the litter box if you are pregnant.

▶ **Consider** biodegradable litter that is made from wheat, pine or other natural products and is available at most pet supply stores. Wear a mask when changing litter to avoid breathing in any dust particles.

Dog waste is not toxic, that is, if you feed your dog non-toxic food. It can be added to your soil or to your non-edible outdoor plants as a beneficial nutrient. Pet enthusiasts can even train their dogs and cats to use the toilet with an inexpensive seat attachment sold at most pet stores! It is easier to train a young dog (or cat) to do new tricks.

Cat waste, on the other hand, should not be used as a fertilizer as it may contain environmentally-resistant eggs of Toxoplasma parasites.

Travel

BEING A GREEN TOURIST

Awakening to the world around us is a beautiful thing. Our path to saving ourselves often takes us into new frontiers.

▶ **Consider** when you find yourself away from home, incorporate your knowledge about how to create essential environments into your stay. Many establishments are making it easier to stay green while traveling. They may provide recycling, chemical-free dry cleaning, organic food, low-flow toilets, energy efficient heat and light, composting and optional laundry.

When you stay in regular establishments, you can make a difference by asking the hotel if they offer any green options or if they plan to do so in the future. As with organic food, when enough customers ask, it will create a demand for greener options.

Have a little less impact and give back a little to the planet in your travels. Of course, that includes enjoying the surroundings yourself. From packing to your mode of transportation, to dining, to your water usage, there is usually a greener choice. Once you save yourself with the ideas in *Essential Environments*, being a green tourist is easy.

CRUISE SHIPS

Cruise ships, just like other structures, are prone to the same types of toxicity. Often referred to as a hotel on water, cruise ships use a tremendous amount of energy and generate a tremendous amount of pollution.

One day while sailing the coastal waters of the United States, I noticed trash floating on top of the water. At first I thought it was just a small amount that had perhaps blown off the deck of another ship. It did not take long for me to realize that this floating landfill was actually miles long. The captain informed me that it was probably dumped from one or several cruise ships. Pollution comes in all kinds of forms and from all kinds of unintended sources.

▶ **Consider**, as with all travel, that choosing companies that practice environmentally-friendly operations is a better selection. Currently there is not one cruise line that is totally eco-friendly; however, leading the charge is Disney Cruise Line. Their website states, "The cast and crew of the two Disney Cruise Ships recognize the value of the ocean as an environment where we are all guests. We will do our best to minimize the impact of this magnificent ecosystem by practicing responsible waste management and stewardship of our ecosystems." Other cruise ship companies are making small eco-friendly changes to their laundry and energy systems, but much, much more could be done.

HOTELS

Hotels are the fourth largest energy consumer in the United States. Toxic solvents and cleaning solutions, disposable amenities, unnecessarily laundered linens and the lack of recycling are pressing issues that need to be addressed.

"Green" hotels or ecotels are a new standard for the hospitality industry. These are hotels that are committing to environmentally-sound practices such as energy and water

As with organic food, when enough customers ask, it will create a demand for greener options.

conservation, waste management, land preservation, environmental training for employees, non-toxic cleaning substances and organic, sustainable food sources.

▶ **Consider** supporting an ecotel for your future travel. There are a few environmentally-sound hotel certification programs within the hotel industry. Although an establishment may not be entirely "green," more and more lodging facilities are trying to improve the situation and need to be supported.

Finding an ecotel may be a bit of a challenge as this is a new groundswell but it will improve as we become more aware consumers. Very few websites are devoted to green lodging but this is changing. Ask the reservationist of the establishment you are thinking of lodging if they are a certified green facility or if they offer patrons a choice of environmentally-friendly services. Even if the hotel where you are staying is not an ecotel, be a green consumer and leave a note for housekeeping that your linens do not need to be changed every day. Conserve your water usage and turn off the lights, heat and air conditioning when you are absent from the room. Call housekeeping and ask that no chemicals be used or sprayed when cleaning your room.

RENTAL CARS

If you have ever rented a car, you have experienced that blast of chemicals that assault you when you open the car door. In an effort to make their cars smell "clean," rental car companies spray car interiors with scented chemicals after each rental.

As the demand for alternate transportation increases, more and more rental car companies will hopefully begin to offer fuel-efficient cars.

▶ **Consider** requesting fragrance-free vehicles when you make your reservation. Fragrance-free rental cars will be just like smoke-free hotel rooms—a result of consumer demand. For now, keep your rental car windows open as much as possible.

Ask for fuel-efficient cars when available since they are a green choice compared to standard cars. EV Car Rentals specializes in renting green vehicles to travelers in 12 cities. (See Sources.)

RESTAURANTS

The Green Restaurant Association (GRA), a national nonprofit organization, provides a convenient way for all sectors of the restaurant industry to become more environmentally sustainable.

Choose restaurants that have both an organic mindset and organic food.

As the demand for organic food increases, restaurants are rushing to offer organic fare. Choose restaurants that have both an organic mindset and organic food. An organic mindset includes making pure, filtered drinking water and ice cubes available, using non-toxic candles, organic flowers, chemical-free soap and cleaning products. Make sure the restaurants you patronize are free of smoke and are fragrance-free. After all, you are at the restaurant to smell, taste and experience your food, not to be assaulted by the stimulation of artificial surroundings.

▶ **Consider** supporting "green" restaurants. Organic Style magazine has a growing list of Reader's Choice Green Restaurants on their website at www.organicstyle.com. To find a green restaurant, visit www.dinegreen.com.

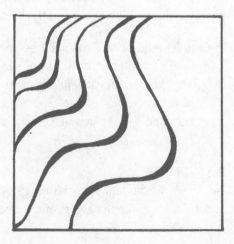

Chapter 3

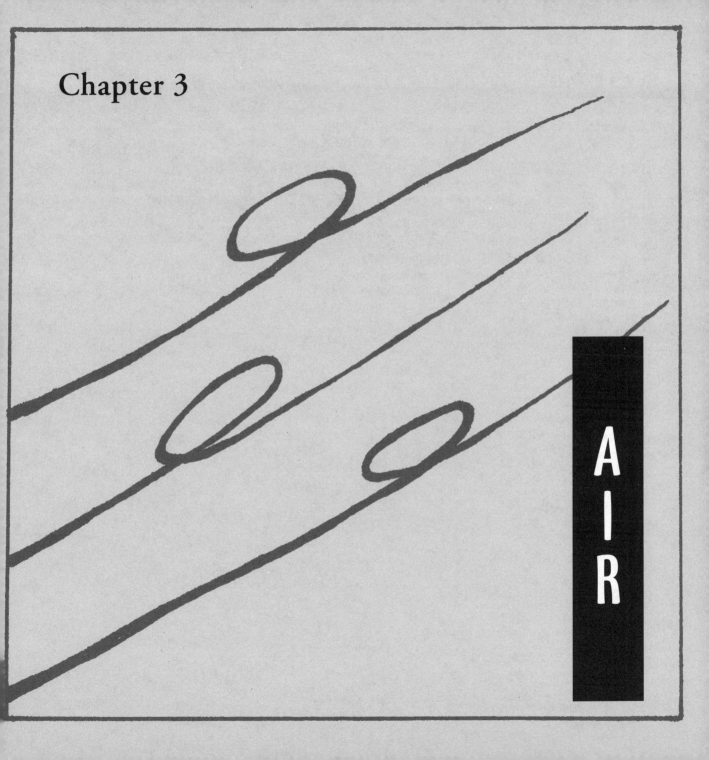

AIR

In This Chapter ⌒ Products and practices relating to the quality of air

Introduction to Air

Another primary ingredient for seeking optimal health and for sustaining life is clean, fresh air. The human body breathes in about 2500 gallons of air every single day. Air, especially clean air, is something that we all certainly take for granted. If you need a quick reminder as to how essential it is, simply try holding your breath for a few seconds!

Air pollution is caused by chemicals, toxic emissions, greenhouse gases, smog, fumes and many other deadly contaminators. Inhalation and skin contact are the two ways through which air pollution enters and invades our bodies. Airborne chemicals come from a variety of sources such as perfumes, smoke, car gases, pet dander, pollen, aerosol sprays, paint, fuel vapors, dry cleaning solvents and plastics, all of which are stored in your body's fatty tissue. More and more people are finding themselves living in areas that actually fail air-quality tests for pollution.

Approximately 38 percent of Americans have some sort of allergy, an abnormal sensitivity to substances called allergens. Many of the most common allergens are found in our air such as pollens, dust mites, molds and animal dander. Even in the solace of nature, finding pure, clean air is becoming increasingly difficult. Unfortunately, in addition to sharing the air with the entire world, we also, share the contaminants that can, but do not have to, consume our right to clean, fresh air.

Considerations for Air

Pause, take a few deep breaths and consider how the quality of your air directly affects your health. Consider that Americans spend 95 percent of their time in man-made environments that are overflowing with poor air quality and potential contaminants. It is easy to become overwhelmed with the idea of cleaning up your air. Again, take a deep breath and consider that your increased awareness will make it easier for you to take the next step. The solutions in this chapter will help you save yourself and your air. Start with one step at a time. You are worth it.

Air Contaminants

AEROSOL SPRAYS

Before grabbing for *any* aerosol spray, consider all the chemicals that they contain and are capable of releasing into your air. Aerosol sprays usually consist of very small droplets of solvent, propellant and active ingredients that are easily absorbed into the nose, throat, lungs and stomach. Just like other harmful chemical forms, these droplets end up contaminating the environment and affecting your body. Through the innocent act of inhalation and the natural absorption process of the skin's pores, we routinely expose ourselves to adverse conditions and situations. Some of the chemicals present in aerosols such as xylene, ketones and aldehydes have been associated with "Sick Building Syndrome"—a very nasty situation.

Included in the aerosol sprays arsenal are hairsprays, adhesives, static eliminators, shaving foam and gel, paints, oven cleaners, furniture polish, deodorants, air fresheners, insect repellant, cleaning products and water repellent sprays.

Aerosol product usage and its ill effects have revealed their true and real potential to cause temporary chest tightness, shortage of breath, headaches, nausea, dizziness, eye and throat irritation, ear infections, diarrhea, and skin rashes. Pregnant women, babies and the elderly are more susceptible to the effects of aerosol sprays.

▶ **Consider** instead alternative methods of product applications such as pump-sprays, roll-ons, liquid and non-aerosol sprays. Pouring, wiping, dusting, and brushing are additional alternatives. Sometimes, all we need to do is use a little more elbow grease and rely less on convenience items. Of course, spending less time cleaning is a natural attraction, but equally important is having the health to enjoy those saved up moments.

In addition to the harmful aspect of aerosol packaging, the majority of **air fresheners** contain chemicals; some even incorporate pesticides into the mix to mask odors in your air. Removing the harmful chemicals in and around your space will eliminate your need for chemical-air fresheners. Whether they are in aerosol cans, plug into a wall outlet or sit on your counter, air fresheners are another source of unnatural chemicals that are brought into your life. We are smarter than this. Use eco- and human-friendly ways to create clean smelling air. See suggestions under Potpourri, Air Purification and Sources. These earth-friendly products may not be the mainstream items you are accustomed to buying; but they are safe, effective and more readily available and reasonably priced than you might think.

Other considerations that can help you make a difference are using **hairspray** pumps instead of sprays, or better yet, trying on a "do" that is hairspray-free. Use **cleaning products** that are in non-aerosol cans, such as paste or wipe-on versions. Use liquid **glues** instead of spray adhesives. Applying **paint** finishes and coatings with a paint brush or

Spending less time cleaning is a natural attraction, but equally important is having the health to enjoy those saved up moments.

sponge as opposed to aerosol spray receptacles is a good choice. Find your creative side while you explore the many different and available **crayons** in the box, nontoxic, that is!

Unless you have become affectionately comfortable with the occasional and embarrassing random sock stuck in your pant leg, these suggestions will prove helpful. To remove **static cling** from clothes without using aerosol products, carefully run a wire clothes hanger over the inside and outside of the garment. If you do not have a wire hanger, dampen your hands and run them over the static fabric where it touches your skin. Hanging a garment near the shower while showering can also eliminate static. Be cling free with your laundry *and* your ideas.

Purchase products that do not require the use of **water-repellent sprays**. Like all aerosol sprays, they are made from chemicals, most of which have not been tested as to long-term effects on humans, yet these chemicals surround us in products we use every day.

Before purchasing aerosol spray products, always pause and ponder their benefits alongside the potential health and environmental risks of using them.

AIR POLLUTANTS

Radon, asbestos, formaldehyde, vinyl and lead are the five most common causes of indoor air pollution. They are present in carpeting, furniture, glues, insulation, siding, cabinetry, kerosene space heaters, paint, and upholstery. Exposure to these and other toxic airborne pollutants such as bacteria, mold and mildew can cause serious health issues.

▶ **Consider** testing your home, office or school for radon. It is a colorless, odorless, tasteless radioactive gas. There are no safe radon levels. Studies show that the better the ventilation, the lower the radon level. When radon is present, air purification units, as well as HEPA vacuum cleaners should be used to remove dust that may contain radioactive particles from radon.

Ask questions about the material substance and content of goods when making home purchases to make sure they do not contain any harmful chemicals. If you have asbestos in your home, contact an expert to determine the appropriate action needed to remove it. Sometimes the removal can be more toxic than just leaving it undisturbed. The risks are relatively small if asbestos is managed and maintained properly.

If you live in a house that was built pre 1978, your paint may contain high levels of lead. Bathtubs manufactured before 1984 may leach lead into bathwater. In most cases, if the paint is in good condition it is not a hazard and to remove it may increase the danger to your family. If you suspect lead hazards in your home, immediately clean up any paint chips and wash floors and painted surfaces with a nontoxic general cleaner. Where children are present, wash their hands frequently, keep play areas clean, and wash toys and stuffed animals regularly. Children can suffer behavior or learning problems due to lead poisoning. For more information on lead hazards and how to treat them, contact the EPA.

Locate a hazardous waste collection site for the proper disposal of existing toxic products. (See Sources for state-by-state locations.) The trip and the bother are worth it in the long run since you will sleep better knowing you are doing the correct thing. Asking your friends and neighbors if you can dispose of their hazardous waste along with yours may inspire them to make a contribution to help build a better world.

Bacteria and mold occur in every space. Bacteria, mold and mildew can result from excess moisture in an environment. In an effort to reduce mold and mildew, fix any leaking pipes or moisture that me by coming into the house from the basement to the attic. Improve the air circulation with fans and place furniture so as to not block air flow. Avoid putting carpet on concrete floors to reduce humidity. Ventilate crawl spaces and attics. Turn on a fan or open a window when showering. Where mold has taken hold, items such as ceiling tiles, carpets, or sheetrock may need to be removed. Most of these basic steps should eliminate and keep bacteria and mold from growing in your space.

CANDLES

Scented candles are emerging as the next addiction in America—they are everywhere. Unfortunately, these aroma-laden wax therapies also emit toxins along with their desirable scents and ambiance. Allergies, asthma, attention deficit, memory loss, neurological damage and other dis-ease symptoms can be traced to scented candles. They also deplete your air of oxygen and fresh air. Simply avoid them. Do not despair—the romance of the candle can still be experienced if you practice safe burning.

▶ **Consider** that the safest and cleanest candles to burn are 100 percent, unscented, color-free beeswax candles with cloth wicks followed by unscented, color-free paraffin or soy candles with cloth wicks.

Pure beeswax and pure soybean candles are made without petroleum additives, are cleaner burning, emit less soot and are longer burning than petroleum-based paraffin candles. These alternative candles are found in a great many natural product and gift

Do not despair—the romance of the candle can still be experienced if you practice safe burning.

stores. Even non-toxic candles deplete your fresh air so make sure to crack a window. Chemically sensitive people should not burn candles or incense.

Essential oil diffusers are a good alternative to burning candles. Essential oils are extracted from plants, fruits and flowers and thus contain the odor or flavor of the plant from which it comes. Diffusers for these oils come in all forms and functions such as lamp ring diffusers, necklace and car diffusers, fan and tea candle diffusers (use only safe tea candles) and diffuser pots. Nebulizing diffusers disperse the oil into the air ionically allowing the oil to be suspended in the air longer. Choose a diffuser that resonates with your style.

CIGARETTES, CIGARS, TOBACCO & SECOND-HAND SMOKE

As per the Surgeon General, first- and second-hand smoke from cigarettes, cigars and pipes is hazardous to your health. Unless you have just crawled out from under a rock, every one of us is aware of these warnings. Enough has been said on this topic already.

▶ **Consider** that you could stop smoking, although it is much easier said than done. Take steps to get help. Wear a patch, use lozenges, or try acupuncture or whatever it takes to rid your life of these toxic substances. You are worth it.

Non-smokers who are exposed to second-hand smoke day after day are at an equal risk of cancer, asthma and heart attacks. You are worth it too.

ELECTRICAL MAGNETIC FIELDS—EMFS

Here is another topic that attracts a great deal of controversy. On one side is the EPA whose job is to warn the public about hazardous environmental situations and; on the other side are the industries that use and produce products that emit EMFs—including the computer, cell phone, appliance and energy industries, and the military. I would certainly not like to deal with this group of opponents.

Environmental stress takes on many forms. It has a vast impact on health even though most often it cannot be seen, heard or felt. Several studies have suggested the link between cancer and exposure to EMFs. The quandary lies in that the EPA cannot label EMFs as a carcinogen because the tests cannot yet demonstrate precisely how this happens or exactly how harmful EMFs really are.

The question remains, can EMFs from power lines, home wiring, airport and military radar, substations, transformers, televisions, computers, lighting fixtures, microwave ovens, refrigerators, electric dishwashers and small electrical appliances cause numerous health problems? Some of the reported health problems include brain tumors, leukemia, birth defects, miscarriages, chronic fatigue, headaches, cataracts, heart problems, stress, nausea, chest pain, forgetfulness, cancer and other health problems. Although numerous studies have produced contradictory results, some experts are convinced that the threat is real. Research does show that low-level magnetic fields and even microwave ovens can disrupt normal brain function.

▶ **Consider** that despite the fact that debates and politics will continue, EMFs will gradually become a very dominant part of our everyday life. For some people they already have. Until safe levels can be determined, consider some of the following solutions for protecting and reducing your exposure to EMFs. The list is lengthy so begin by choosing those to which you can easily adapt. Later on, you can incorporate the rest into your lifestyle as your health dictates.

Until safe levels can be determined, consider some of the following solutions for protecting and reducing your exposure to EMFs.

Be sure to sit at least three feet, preferably six feet, away from electrical appliances, such as televisions, lamps, toasters, computers, refrigerators, etc. Especially when sleeping, make sure that any electronic device is at least three feet away from your body. EMFs are significantly less when they are three or more feet away from an electrical source. Do not use electric blankets or sleep on a water bed. Eliminate electrical wires running under the bed. Avoid sleeping in the room where the electricity physically enters into the home. Computer shielding products and low-radiation CRT (cathode ray tube) display screens are available to reduce EMF exposure.

Use battery-powered clocks versus electrically powered ones. Old-fashioned wind-up watches emit less EMFs than a quartz-analog watch that pulsates EMFs along the body's acupuncture meridians. Electric razors and hair dryers are sources of EMFs. Avoid using hair dryers on children to protect them from the high EMF exposure so close to their developing brain. Small adjustments such as air-dried hair or shaving with an old-fashioned style razor can help reduce overexposure of EMFs on a daily level.

Avoid living in homes that are near a power line, substations, power-generating stations or transformers (a difficult task as they are located in almost every neighborhood). Also, be alert to military and airport radar systems, both of which emit EMFs.

To find out how you can reduce your exposure to EMFs from cell phones, see Sources under Wireless Phones. Telephones and telephone answering machines emit strong EMFs, especially from headsets and handsets. The dilemma is that we, as individuals, are similar to magnets that attract this harmful field through our accessories and surroundings.

Microwave ovens give off EMFs. Recent Russian studies have shown that normal microwave cooking converts food protein into carcinogenic substances. Use conventional cooking skills, appliances and utensils to prepare food. Traditional ovens give off EMFs also, but do not alter the food. Fluorescent bulbs give off more EMFs than incandescent bulbs. Dimmer and three-way electrical switches give off more EMFs than single on-off switches.

If you want to determine the amount of EMFs radiating outside or inside your home, office or school or from a particular appliance, you can rent or purchase a Gauss meter, an instrument which measures the strength of magnetic fields. Be sure to follow the exact directions for measuring the EMFs. An economical pen-sized meter is available for use so you can determine the level of EMFs that are present in your home and work environments. (See Sources.)

FRAGRANCES, PERFUMES & COLOGNES

Once upon a time fragrance was made from distilled flowers. Today it is made with synthetic chemicals. There are no governing agencies that identify and implement any guidelines or regulations for fragrances. The chemicals used in fragrances are not required to be screened by or to be regulated by any authority. Synthetic fragrances are one of the five major contributors to indoor air pollution. Ninety-five percent of chemicals used in fragrances are synthetic compounds derived from petroleum. Over 85 percent of fragrance ingredients have never been tested for human toxicity.

Fragrances routinely and, sad to admit, legally include ingredients which are known toxins and sensitizers capable of causing cancer, birth defects, central nervous system disorders, allergic reactions, headaches, disorientation, nausea, anxiety, depression, mood swings, lethargy, ear pain, dizziness, vertigo, coughing, seizures, rashes, eczema, joint pain, hypertension, swollen lymph glands and fatigue—just to mention a few! One may wonder if multiple sclerosis, Parkinson's disease, lupus and Alzheimer's disease, all neurological disorders, could be caused by exposure to neurotoxic chemicals.

Fragrances are ever increasingly being added to an endless parade of products to the point of desensitizing our olfactory nerves, thereby causing a loss of smell. Fabric softeners, detergents, candles, hygienic products, foods, oils, solvents, garbage bags, diapers, kitty litter and inks are just a few products that have fragrances. Ann Dermatol Vernereol wrote in the French Toxicology Journal, "Perfumes may produce toxic and more often allergic respiratory disorders (asthma), as well as neurological disorders." One out of every five asthmatics experiences an attack as a result of exposure to perfume. When exposed to them in small spaces, perfumes are the leading cause of headaches.

Most of us have had that unpleasant experience of being in an elevator or restaurant with a person who reeks of perfume. Most likely they have reapplied the fragrance several times because they can no longer smell the fragrance since their olfactory sensory system is so damaged. Remember, what smells wonderful to some can be offensive to others. It seems that our obsession with odor elimination and other personal preferences have in the end rendered us desensitized with health problems as a consequence.

The Americans with Disabilities Act guarantees access for the disabled to public places like institutions, medical offices, retail stores and others. Multiple Chemical Sensitivity / Environmental Illness is recognized as a disability. For that reason, fragrance is a "barrier to access" for the life sustaining activity of breathing and is prohibited in public places. The difficulty in enforcing fragrance bans in public places is evident in the intolerable air quality surrounding the perfume/cosmetic counters in department stores. This is a category about which I could write an entire book, but I will sum it up by saying that most fragrances are toxic and it is best to avoid them.

Most fragrances are toxic and it is best to avoid them.

▶ **Consider**, strongly consider, eliminating perfume from your life. If you are resisting this consideration, you may be one of the countless people that have become addicted to these poisons. Instead of chemical-laden synthetic perfumes, take a bottle of fragrance-free lotion and add a few drops of your favorite essential oil. Use this lotion as a scent when you are not going to be in public places or around those in your home that are sensitive to fragrance. Be considerate of yourself and your coworkers when you select a product that contains a scent.

Use environment- and human-friendly products for household cleaners and cosmetics that are fragrance-free. A few companies are leading the effort to use only essential oils extracted from plants that have been grown under certifiably organic conditions. (See Bath & Beauty Products in the Earth Chapter.)

Be careful of fragrance terminology. Unscented is not fragrance-free. "Unscented" products usually use a "masking fragrance" to cover up the original fragrance. Avoid all scented and unscented products and those that list "fragrance" as an ingredient, unless it states that the fragrance is derived from an essential oil.

Essential oils are oils extracted from plants, fruits and flowers. Make sure you are not allergic to a particular essential oil before using it. Even though they are natural, if you are allergic to citrus, you will likely be allergic to lemon and other citrus essential oils. A good example is poison ivy. It is 100 percent natural, but can cause an unpleasant reaction when it comes in contact with your skin.

INDUSTRIAL AIR POLLUTION

This topic and others like global warming is complex and can prove to be overwhelming to the individual. Power plants are the nation's second-largest source of nitrogen-oxide pollution after automobiles. Exposure to industrial emissions of nitrogen oxide, sulfur dioxide, carbon dioxide, and mercury can cause birth defects, cancer, developmental delays and learning disorders. Public awareness and community participation are the two most important steps toward change. This knowledge will help you to support politicians who are advocates of clean technology. Ignoring industrial pollution brings the inevitable burden of clean up—health related, financial, and environmental clean-up is accelerating as the years progress.

For those of you who understand that industrial air pollution directly affects your health and lifestyle, form a coalition or work through a liaison to halt or at least to discuss future guidelines to prevent further damage. If you work every day in an industrial environment or live near or next to such sites, these issues are indeed essential to address.

Sadly, most politicians and corporations only move toward cleaning up and preventing pollution when they see that the benefits of controlling it exceed the costs to do so. The purpose of the Clean Air Act has been delayed and weakened by many power companies, lawyers and politicians who refuse and resist putting health and safety above money and profit. Over the last 20 years, power companies have used their political clout and to diminish the efforts of the EPA to reduce toxic emissions. Millions of tons of harmful pollutants are being released into the air from power plants violating the Clean Air Act. Although pollution-controlling scrubbers on power plants can cut emissions up to 95 percent they can be costly. If only the cost of acid-rain, smog and poor health had a price tag.

▶ **Consider** that your vote matters. Discover which candidates and organizations are environmentally-conscientious, active, and committed and then support them.

MAGAZINES

The fragrance industry is a big dollar and *scents* business. Colognes, perfumes, and the gamut of aromatherapy products advertised in magazines are usually accompanied with a scented card, a kind of "up your nose" instead of "in your face" advertising! There is nothing romantic about the chemicals contained in perfume. The fragrance industry has brainwashed us into believing that our natural scent needs to be masked with toxic chemicals. We have been lulled by the dreaminess of illusion and passion that scents can unleash and create. Wake up and refuse to smell the toxicity!

Fragrance bans are greeted with great resistance and reticence by publications and their advertisers. They are both intrinsically positioned to make huge profits on these harmful, chemical-laden and typically unregulated products. We are, without a doubt, much smarter than to buy mass marketing techniques and products that stink! (See Fragrance for reasons on how and why to eliminate these chemicals from your life.)

▶ **Consider** canceling magazine subscriptions that include fragrance-scented cards. Why invite these chemicals into your home or office? Write to the magazine editors and tell them your preference for fragrance-free reading. Your active protest, manifested as a refusal to continue your subscription, will remind them that pleasing their customers is vitally important to profitability.

As of January 1992, California passed a law that scented advertisements in printed material such as newspapers, magazines and periodicals shall be enclosed in a sealant designed to protect the consumer from inadvertent exposure. The United States Postal Service also regulates fragrance advertising samples. Unfortunately, this has not been enough to keep the smell out of our reading material, mail and nose.

NOISE POLLUTION

Hearing is fundamental to language, communication, socialization and pleasure. Over 36 million Americans suffer from the negative effects of noise pollution. Almost everyone has experienced noise in certain environments that is well above the normal limit.

▶ **Consider** protecting yourself from noise pollution by carrying a pair of earplugs to use in public places where you cannot control the volume—such as inside airplanes, movie theatres, concerts and indoor sporting events. Noise levels in a workplace, exceeding 90 decibels (db) are mandated by law for hearing protection. Avoid noise-polluted places. Check the volume of your headset. If you are experiencing hearing loss, have your hearing tested by an audiologist. Take a quiet drive or walk in the countryside and just listen to the sounds that normally elude us in the noisy cities. Once

The fragrance industry has brainwashed us into believing that our natural scent needs to be masked with toxic chemicals.

you realize what you are missing or not hearing, you will want to "change your tune" or at least lower its volume!

PET LITTER

Many pet litters are prepared with chemical additives for controlling odor. For the most part, litters are made with clay that is not easily decomposed. A simple step such as changing the brand of the litter you purchase can reduce chemical exposure for you and your pets.

▶ **Consider** using a natural substance for pet litter, such as wheat or pine chips or pieces. Both neutralize odors naturally, create less dust and are biodegradable. Sold at most pet stores, these healthy alternatives to clay-based litters will be a treat for your pets. (See Pet Litter in the Earth chapter.)

POTPOURRI

Fragrance added to potpourri is another portal that allows chemicals to enter our lives. Potpourri, by definition, is a mixture of various scents used to perfume, not contaminate a room. When was the last time, if ever, that you saw an all inclusive ingredient list on a package of potpourri?

▶ **Consider** instead that you can make your own potpourri, one that is natural and non-toxic. A few suggestions include putting dried rose petals in a bowl and sprinkling a few drops of a floral essential oil, such as geranium or lavender, over them. Place some dried orange slices in a dish with a few drops of lemon, orange or tangerine essential oil. Put some herbs or pine cones in a bowl with a few drops of your favorite essential oil, such as eucalyptus or bergamot. Refresh when needed.

Here is a safe way to clear your air of odors, especially moldy odors in the bathroom. Cut an orange in half, scoop out the pulp, fill each half with table salt and place in the bathroom. Refresh when the salt hardens.

For a safe, easy way to fill your space with a wonderful aroma is to put 4-6 cups of water in a saucepan. Add a chopped apple or a chopped orange with the rind. Stir in 2 teaspoons of cinnamon and 1 teaspoon of ground cloves. Bring to a boil, reduce heat and simmer until the water has almost evaporated, making sure the pan does not boil dry. As the mixture simmers it will emit a spicy, home-baked aroma.

SUN RAYS

Common knowledge tells us that harmful ultra violet (UV) rays from the sun can cause short- and long-term injury including sun-induced skin aging and skin cancers.

▶ **Consider** wearing UV protective clothing like brimmed hats or shirts when in the sun. Several companies make sun-sensitive and sun-sensible clothing. It is a great way to protect yourself from the sun.

Use an effective, fragrance-free sunscreen that contains both UVA and UVB filters. Take extra care with infants and children by applying and reapplying sunscreen often. Limit children's sun exposure and keep infants shaded from sunrays. Wear sunglasses. Sit in the shade. Moderation and common sense are the best guidelines concerning sun exposure and sensitivity.

Air Purification

AIR FILTRATION & PURIFICATION

Not much can compare to an exhilarating burst of fresh air, be it warm or cold.

We often forget that just like food and water, air is made up of energy. When this energy is clean and pure, it supports health and well-being. When air is polluted, it breaks down our health and causes dis-ease. The United States House of Representatives and the Environmental Protection Agency (EPA) state that indoor air pollution is our number one environmental health problem today. The fact that 90 percent of colds are caught indoors and 10 percent are caught outdoors exemplifies this point.

▶ **Consider** as a first line of defense removing and eliminating the sources of air pollution in your environment. Some common, everyday offenders are cleaning products, pesticides, plastics and synthetic fibers, particleboard furniture and cabinets, fragrances, carpeting, drapes, scented candles, scented products, pet odors, gas appliances and heaters, and other seemingly harmless items made from petrochemicals.

Next, open your windows to ventilate the space. Not much can compare to an exhilarating burst of fresh air, be it warm or cold. The sultry caress of a warm breeze or the ruddy blast of a bitterly cold wind will affect your physical well-being while simultaneously lifting your spirits. An easy and economical way to rid your space of unwanted odors and fumes more quickly is to place a window fan in a centrally located window facing out. Just like in built-in exhausts found in kitchens and bathrooms, this will create an exhaust for your living space.

The third consideration for cleaner air is plants. The National Aeronautics and Space Administration (NASA) states that common houseplants *remove* pollutants during their natural process of photosynthesis. Plants can be very effective in removing low-level gases such as carbon dioxide, formaldehyde, carbon monoxide, cigarette smoke, benzene and smog. Plants such as bamboo palms, dracaena palms, aloe plants, philodendrons, spider plants and schleffleras make good air filters. Depending on the number of pollutants present, two good sized plants can purify the air in a 10- by 10-foot room.

If your air quality remains at a poor level, select an air purification or filtration system for your home or work space. Purification methods neutralize and remove airborne particles through ion and ozone generators. Filtration methods, such as High Efficiency Particulate Air filters (HEPA) and carbon media, push air through a filter in an effort to trap airborne contaminants. Other air cleaners include ultraviolet (UV) light, molecular absorption and lava rocks. Each uses a different process and each is capable of filtering different particles out of the air.

The information available on air purification systems can be varied and conflicting. The severity of your air quality will determine the steps you need to take. Listed below are the types of air purification and filtration technology. Unfortunately, no single method does it all. The contaminants in the air are small, medium and large particulate, bacteria, viruses, fungi, mold, gases and odors. Keep this in mind when you select a purification system, because its effectiveness results from proper identification of the contaminant being addressed.

Once your air cleaning requirements and the size of the space you wish to treat has been determined, choose a machine to purify your air. Often, machines combine technologies to better filter the air. Quality equipment will last longer and will usually perform better than less expensive models so invest once instead of spending twice. (See Sources.)

Ion generation. Air is made up of energy—molecules, to be exact. Clean air is comprised of a balanced positive (proton) and negative (electron) nucleus charge. Pollution disrupts this balance and causes more positive ions to be created, thereby outnumbering the electrons. However, do not be confused since positive in this case is a bad thing; conversely, negative is a good thing. Simply, ion generators give off a negative charge to the positively charged airborne dust particles making them heavy enough to drop out of the air.

Human health is compromised when an abundance of positive ions are present in the air. Many regions around the globe experience debilitating positive-ion winds such as the Santa Ana winds, Chinook winds, and Mistral winds.

More negative ions are generated in nature than in our man-made environments. For example, a waterfall generates 100,000 ions per cubic centimeter and a home's interior only generates 0—500 ions per cubic centimeter. Lightning generates 100,000,000 ions per cubic centimeter. Hopefully, you have felt the healing effects of these negative ions while sitting by the ocean, walking in a mountain forest or after a lightning storm.

▶ **Consider** that research shows that negative ions can improve overall health, reduce depression, headaches, allergies, and asthma, give you more energy, help you sleep better and enable you to feel less anxious. You do not have to wait for lightning to strike; there are safer ways in which to alter your indoor air, *in a negative way!* You can create more negative ions in your man-made environment with a machine called an ionizer, sometimes called an electron generator or negative ion generator. Ionizers come in room and personal-use sizes. Select an ionizer that is the correct size for balancing the charges in your designated indoor area.

Once the airborne contaminants attach to the dust particles through the ionization process, they gain added weight and fall to the floor or surrounding surfaces. Make certain that you place the machine in the middle of the room so the pollutants can be easily cleaned, vacuumed and disposed of properly.

Negative ion generators neutralize most airborne particles including allergens and irritants but do not neutralize gases or various odors. A machine that combines ion generation and low-level ozone generation is best if these particles and gases are present. The following are the various purifying and filtering options available for your consideration.

Ozone generation. Ozone occurs in nature and is responsible for neutralizing gases and odors. Ozone is the layer of the upper atmosphere that protects us from ultra violet rays. People mistakenly confuse ozone with smog. Ozone is not a by-prod-

Hopefully, you have felt the healing effects of these negative ions while sitting by the ocean, walking in a mountain forest or after a lightning storm.

uct of automobile exhaust. Ozone is created when the ultraviolet rays from the sun strike the hydrocarbons from auto exhaust. When pollution gets high, ozone helps oxidize and clear the air. Because ozone is more easily detected than hydrocarbons it is used as a reference point for the level of pollution.

Ozone is also created when oxygen is released from plant life and combines with the sun's ultraviolet rays. This process is accomplished by binding a third oxygen atom to the two already existing atoms of normal oxygen. When the third atom detaches, pollutants are oxidized. Sorry for the science lesson, but there is much confusion over ozone, natures natural oxidizer.

Closer to the earth, electrical currents such as those in lightning, transform oxygen into ozone. Low levels of machine generated ozone can be used indoors to reproduce the process of nature's greatest purifier and oxidizer.

▶ **Consider** investing in an ozone generator or an ozonation device to sterilize and remove odors, bacteria, viruses, fungus, mold and gases that are present in your air. Ozone generators do not eliminate airborne dust particles as well as negative ion generators. Therefore, many air purifiers combine the two technologies, ionization and ozonation as an ideal solution for removing micro organisms and airborne bacteria, gases and odors.

For those still concerned about the level of ozone output from an ozone generator compare these parts per million (ppm) for ozone that occurs indoors and outdoors. The range in which ozone occurs in a healthy outdoor setting is .02—.05 ppm. Typical smog is .5 ppm. In nearly all indoor environments with open window air circulation the ozone level is .001 ppm. The average output from an ozone generator is .005 ppm, the same level it occurs in nature. Room coverage varies with machines. Make sure when considering an ozone generator that the output covers the space you wish to purify.

Electrostatic precipitators. Electrostatic precipitators are used primarily for controlling industrial air pollution and can be found on large power plants, cement plants, incinerators, and boiler emissions. It is a highly efficient way to remove large particles, heavy metals, mists, dioxins, and fumes from process gas streams.

This technology, sometimes called an electrostatic or electronic particulate filter, is also available for home air purifiers. The magnetic static connection is used to neutralize and collect particles. Models usually collect particles inside the machine on panels that need to be cleaned often.

▶ **Consider** that although these filters can remove up to 95 percent of large particulates, including dust, dirt and smoke, they do not remove *all* gases and odors and *do not* oxidize mold, viruses or fungus. Unlike other purifiers, this technology only filters air that passes through the unit. Electrostatic air purifiers that have an ultraviolet light are better at killing viruses and bacteria.

If these reasons comprise a drawback or a concern to your intended results, consider other air purifying technologies.

Ultra violet light. This type of purification disinfects air when it is exposed to ultra violet (UV) light. The Federal Trade Commission (FTC) states that the potential effect of UV light on bacteria depends upon a number of factors—the wattage of the light, the distance of the organism from the light, and the length of exposure under the light. Bacterial spores would require a relatively long time under the light for it to have a killing effect. Most household air cleaners move air too quickly to provide adequate exposure time for such an assassination.

To further restore or maintain the air quality in a space, have the heating ducts professionally cleaned.

▶ **Consider** investigating the above factors if UV light is an alternative for sterilizing your air. UV light has been successfully used to disinfect the air in hospitals and manufacturing plants. It is especially effective when installed in building ventilation systems where there is contamination from moisture condensation from air-conditioning systems.

Filtration. Air filtration simply pushes air through a filter to remove airborne particles. There are several concerns with filtration systems. The air that does not flow into the system goes untreated. There is the added maintenance of remembering to purchase and replace filters. Sometimes there are contamination problems when filters are not replaced as suggested. Over the life of an air filter, purchasing replacement filters can add up to more than the initial costs of more expensive and effective systems.

▶ **Consider** that air filters are usually less expensive than the alternatives mentioned above. Remember to change the filters according to the manufacturer's instructions thus preventing an air filter from becoming a breeding ground for bacteria and mold.

Of all the filters, High Efficiency Particulate Air (HEPA) filters are the most effective for removing particles and some bacteria. The next most effective filters are foam and fiber filters. Carbon media or activated charcoal filters are less satisfactory in filtering dust particles as well, but they are effective in removing gases and odors.

To further restore or maintain the air quality in a space, have the heating ducts professionally cleaned. The National Air Duct Cleaners Association (nadac.com) suggests that debris and dust can become lodged in the ducts causing poor air quality in a home or office. Filters on a furnace can be upgraded to a pleated filter that captures smaller particles than standard filters. The key is to change them regularly—every couple of months.

Lava rocks. All odors are positively-charged gases that float in the air like dust particles. All-natural, odorless, nontoxic volcanic crystals called lava rock contain a negative charge. The crystals act like a magnet attracting and absorbing all odors, keeping the air clean and fresh smelling.

▶ **Consider** that if it is odors alone that you want to rid from your air, The Gonzo Corporation makes a product called the Odor Eliminator, which are lava rock crystals in mesh bags. They remove unpleasant cooking odors from kitchens and smoke odors from cigars, cigarettes, fireplaces and wood-burning stoves. They will also remove pet odors from litter boxes and pet accidents, musty odors in basements and garages and odors in closets. Odor Eliminators can keep car, truck, boat and RV interiors smelling fresh and clean. This is a good idea when you know the source of contamination such as a pipe smoker or a pet. This option allows removal of the evidence instead of the culprit such as a family member or pet!

Simply place the mesh bag in any area where an odor exists. In eight to twelve hours all odors are usually gone. After ten months, leave the mesh bag in the sunlight for six hours. This exposure will recharge the crystals making them an economical odor-controlling tool that can be used repeatedly. (See Sources.)

An inexpensive solution for removing odors from a musty basement or stuffy attic is to place a bag of lava or activated charcoal, purchased at a hardware store, behind a 2- by 2-foot box fan running on low speed. The suction of the fan keeps the bag in place while providing circulation of the lave rocks or charcoal.

Molecular absorption. A molecular absorber, another odor control device, removes odors and locks them into a container filled with tiny blue pellets. They are sold in 16- and 32-ounce containers and eliminate odors including fumes and gases. However, they do not eliminate dust particulate from the air.

▶ **Consider** a molecular absorber as an option if odors are your concern. Molecular absorbers do not use electricity, are nontoxic and have biodegradable pellets which need to be replaced when they turn pink. (See Sources.)

BIRDS TO THE RESCUE

The coal miners took canaries down into the mines and used the bird's physical reactions as warning signals to indicate that deadly gases were present. Today, in biochemical warfare the military uses chickens to warn them of airborne toxic chemicals. These are extremely dangerous situations but ours is no less serious. Even though we live in the midst of deadly chemicals day after day, no warning system exists to protect us. Can you imagine boarding a bus or the subway with a caged chicken aboard? Not likely.

Can you imagine boarding a bus or the subway with a caged chicken aboard?

▶ **Consider** that by incorporating some of these ideas for protecting and improving your air quality will reduce and at times deter the exposure to these toxic chemicals that constantly attack your bodies' immune system.

TREES & PLANTS

Trees and plants just keep on giving. They are the air purifiers of the earth. Trees, along with their beauty and stature, are continuously filtering pollutants out of the air so we can breathe easier. Green foliage is easy on the eyes and easy on the lungs.

▶ **Consider** planting a tree or adopting a few house plants to increase indoor oxygen and decrease the effects of airborne contaminants. It is said that a tree never really stops growing—what a beautiful sentiment to apply to our own lives. Thank your favorite tree today.

Machines & Equipment Concerning Air

AUTOMOBILES & TRANSPORTATION

Driving a car is absolutely the single most polluting thing that almost all of us do; and, unfortunately, we do it almost every day! Fossil fuel combustion from motor vehicles, airplanes, recreational vehicles and more, generate 80 percent of the nation's pollution. The emitted gases are the main components relating to the causes of acid rain and global warming.

The problem with transportation pollution is that it is connected to so many other aspects. For example, roads, parking lots and other infrastructures for cars can use one-third to two-thirds of a municipality's land depending upon the population. The more artificial our surroundings become the more artificial our air becomes. Progress always carries with it the innate quality of continual maintenance of its by-products. Asphalt and concrete displace both man and nature as it contributes to pollution and soil erosion.

The good news is that the available technology is geared toward more environmentally-friendly modes of transportation that are less dependent on oil. Several auto makers are answering the demand from consumers for alternatives to gas guzzling and polluting cars. Until we can all embrace cars that use cleaner alternative fuel, all of our combined steps to reduce our personal car usage will help.

▶ **Consider** that you could reduce your transportation usage and your waistline by walking whenever possible. More than 25 percent of Americans car trips are a mile or less. Use public transportation—pick up a schedule of your area's trains, subways, or bus. Plan your trips and errands so that you travel the least amount of miles.

Check into the *Commuters Choice* programs offered by the Environmental Protection Agency and the U.S. Department of Transportation. *Commuters Choice* reduces pollution, reduces traffic congestion and conserves energy through businesses that sponsor employee initiatives for greener commuting. Employers benefit through lowered costs and taxes and employee benefit through savings and incentives.

Ride a bike. Many municipalities are making available fleets of donated or refurbished bikes for environmentally-friendly transportation for city dwellers who want a bike for a day or to run errands. Most programs are free. You can visit www.ibike.org/encouragement/freebike.htm to see if your town has such a program. Perhaps you can help start a program in your own town! Keep a bike at your workplace to use instead of your car for errands. Kits are available to turn your bicycle into an Xtracycle, a conventional bike with an extended frame, making it possible to carry groceries, coolers and kayaks! Human-powered vehicles (HPV) and are also an option for car-less travel. (See Sources) The Better World club is a roadside-assistance program for eco-conscious travelers. They provide cars *and bicycles* with similar services as other motor clubs, but a portion of their revenues are donated to cleaning up the environment.

Share rides with people in your community, neighborhood, or workplace—make new friends—break old thinking patterns! Visit www.carpool.net to find people in your area that are willing to carpool.

Join a car-sharing co-op as a great way to divide the cost of owning a car between a group of people. Car-sharing has many benefits—financially, socially and environmentally. To find a car-sharing network near you, visit www.carsharing.net. An organization called Zipcar makes cars available in Boston, New York and Washington, DC. Members can reserve the use of a car for an hour or more. Visit www.zipcar.com.

Drive your vehicle at a moderate speed. One second of high-powered driving can emit nearly as much carbon monoxide as a half hour of normal driving. The faster you travel, the greater the emissions. Keep your vehicle in good running condition. Change your oil as scheduled at a location that recycles their oil. Keep your tires properly inflated. Buy low-rolling-resistance (LLR) replacement tires that can improve a vehicle's fuel economy. A properly maintained vehicle will emit ten times *less* emissions than a poorly maintained one.

Turn your car off if it is going to be idling for more than 30 seconds. After that, the engine consumes more gas to idle than it does to restart it. When possible on hot days, park in the shade, garage or underground parking to keep your car cool.

Trade in your gas guzzler for a more eco-friendly car such as a hybrid car. Hybrid vehicles combine gasoline with electric motors and rechargeable batteries that are recharged while you drive. They use less gas and emit fewer toxins than traditional cars. In addition to hybrids, future cars will include high-tech diesels, electric and fuel cell models. The range of fuel-efficient and flexible fuel model cars is expanding and will eventually include zero emission vehicles (ZEVs) for a clean-air choice.

One of the clean burning alternative fuels is biodiesel. It is produced from a sustainable resource, usually soybean oil and emits less toxicity when used as fuel. It does not contain petroleum, is biodegradable, nontoxic, and essentially free of sulfur and aro-

The range of fuel-efficient and flexible fuel model cars is expanding and will eventually include zero emission vehicles (ZEVs) for a clean-air choice.

matics. Biodiesel can be used in existing diesel engines with little or no modifications. Car manufacturers are also working to make commercially viable and safe hydrogen powered full cell vehicles, which use hydrogen to produce electricity, with water as a byproduct. Even though they face considerable challenges in mainstreaming these technologies, alternative fuels are necessary in order to create a cleaner environment, a more stable climate and lower public health costs.

Some eco-conscious companies are experimenting with these low-polluting engines by using them in a few urban buses and commercial truck fleets. UPS currently operates over 1,000 natural gas vehicles and is testing hydrogen fuel cell trucks.

Buy local products when possible in order to help reduce tens of millions of gallons of diesel fuel created by delivery trucks. If possible, consolidating many orders into one can realistically impact the emissions saved by decreasing the number of trips needed to ship your freight.

Keep your car windows open or at least cracked when you're on the road. Studies have shown that the air quality inside a car can be much more toxic than air outside. Especially when following another car or truck. Children are at risk of inhaling toxic diesel emissions on school busses. Visit the National Resources Defense Council website, www.ndrc.org for suggestions on how to improve this hazard.

HOME & YARD POWER EQUIPMENT

In the United States, we have 100 million pieces of yard equipment (lawn mowers, snow blowers, leaf blowers and weed trimmers) that emit toxic fumes. The American Lung Association claims that it takes 17 cars to make as much smog as one leaf blower. An additional 17 million gallons of fuel is spilled each year when users refill their outdoor power equipment. Yard equipment generates 5 percent of the nation's air pollution. You would have to drive 100 miles to create the same amount of air pollution as one hour of gas-powered lawn mower.

Fortunately, by the year 2007 yard equipment manufacturers will be required to comply with the EPA's new emissions standards that include catalytic converters and noise pollution reduction.

▶ **Consider** that if you have a small yard, you can mow the lawn with a human-powered lawn mower—get a little exercise while you cut your grass. Or use an electric-powered mower to eliminate odors, emissions and noise. Cordless, battery-driven or electric mowers are more convenient and less expensive to maintain because they do not require gas, oil, spark plugs or tune-ups. An emission-free, battery-powered riding mower can run up to three hours on one charge.

Be adventurous and convert all or part of your yard into indigenous, perennial plantings that take less water, and maintenance. Planting ground cover in more areas of your yard can cut down on the gas and chemicals used to maintain grass. Rake leaves by hand instead of using a leaf blower. Raking can provide a very calming repetition of motion punctuated by the soft smell of damp soil and leaves. Connecting with your yard can help you determine your maintenance needs.

Some vacuum cleaners, although not gasoline-driven, can put as much pollution back into the air as they collect from the floor. HEPA filter vacuum cleaners filter out more airborne particles than regular vacuum cleaners.

SPORT VEHICLES

This is a topic that could transport a lot of heat in my direction. Gas-operated sport vehicles like personal water crafts (PWCs), snowmobiles and all-terrain vehicles (ATVs) contribute to our air and water pollution. To make matters worse, the loud engines and fumes, a double whammy, disturbs wildlife habitats. How amenable you are to these considerations will determine the extent of realistically creating an essential, sustainable environment. Amenities are not entitlements when they become detrimental to our well-being and trespass on the world around us.

There is a continuing debate on the pollution of our national parks, country sides and waterways from gas-powered sport vehicles. Like so many other topics, its resolution often comes down to money. Snowmobiles alone generate an annual $7 billion industry. The people who benefit from the sales of these machines and accessories certainly do not want to ban them, even at the cost of polluting our national parks.

It is in situations like these, where we attempt to make a choice based on nostalgia, tradition, satisfaction, profit, security and propriety, that we must be patient and understanding with ourselves. Little by little, even in unfamiliar territory, we can commit to some positive concessions for the wellness of all. Trust yourself. Your decisions could be healthy ones.

The good news is that as gas-powered engines for automobiles become cleaner, stricter requirements for other machines will follow suit.

▶ **Consider** becoming part of the solution by cleaning up our air, not just in national parks but in your own backyard. Unfortunately, gas-powered sports vehicles just add to air and water pollution. If you can not give up these activities completely, try reducing your usage.

The good news is that as gas-powered engines for automobiles become cleaner, stricter requirements for other machines will follow suit. Dream of the day where we will have quieter, park-friendly, people-friendly, eco-friendly recreational vehicles.

WIRELESS PHONES

Wireless phones emit low-level radio wave radiation—also known as radio frequency (RF) radiation. The safety of wireless phones is another widely debated subject. Some link the radiation from wireless phones to brain tumors, headaches, sleeping disorders and memory loss. Experts to date have found no evidence supporting these claims. In view of the fact that wireless phones have been in use for only a relatively short time, any valid or scientific tests administered to determine their effects on the human body have limitations. It makes sense that although the RF fields from wireless phones are below guideline levels, there is a reason why these guideline levels were set in the first place. Continued research is needed to examine the long-term, harmful potential of RF radiation on humans.

▶ **Consider** that although wireless phone safety accessories alone cannot protect you, they can reduce your exposure to RF radiation. Use an RF-safe ear piece or headset, RF-safe earbuds, and RF-safe pocket, purse or belt shield which are designed to deflect RF radiation. Use RF-approved hands-free devices in your car and an RF approved car antenna. Use land-line phones when possible. By limiting your wireless phone conversations, you can decrease your exposure to harmful radiation.

Public Places

PUBLIC PLACES

You cannot control the air in a public place. You can be in close proximity to those who are wearing toxic chemicals ranging from fabric softener to perfume. In addition, due to the demands for energy conservation, public places are often super-insulated, airtight places that do not allow the pollution to escape.

Airplanes can be especially harmful because everybody from infants to the elderly and the infirm are crammed into a small space with a closed circulating air supply.

Some restaurant owners are now requesting that their patrons not wear perfume or cologne when dining with them. Whether the establishment requires it or not, it is a good idea not to wear these harmful chemicals for the benefit of all involved—at home or in public.

▶ **Consider** that when you remove the chemicals from your world, it will be a beacon for others to do the same. (See Fragrances.) For now, just save yourself by refusing to use common scents!

When a person exudes chemicals on an airline or in any space-challenged public place, move your seat when possible or leave the area. Using a personal negative-ion generating air purifier can help in these situations.

Avoid these toxic areas whenever possible, or at least go outdoors as soon as possible as an antidote to stale indoor air.

AIRPLANE CABIN AIR

Suddenly you smell toxic cleaning and laundry products, air fresheners, lingering perfume and/or cigarette smoke. What do you do?

Controversy over airplane cabin air has been debated for decades. Since the early 1990s, Flight attendants, pilots and passengers have complained to the airlines and airline manufacturers regarding the harmful health effects they believe stem from repeated exposure to contaminated cabin air. Memory loss, respiratory problems, allergic reactions, flu-like symptoms, and neurological damage are some of the symptoms that have been reportedly caused by poor cabin air quality. Although older models of airplanes provide 100% fresh air to the aircraft cabin, newer models of jet aircraft provide up to 50% re-circulated air. Recycled air systems allow newer model aircraft to conserve fuel. It is the effectiveness of these filtration systems that is often the focus of debate on cabin air quality. Currently, the FAA does not require airlines to use air filters.

Consumer complaints and pending lawsuits over cabin air quality will build momentum for the Federal Aviation Association (FAA) to set air quality testing and standards.

▶ **Consider** using a personal negative-ion generating air purifier when traveling. They are very small and are worn around the neck. When using one, I definitely notice the difference in how I feel after flying. Today I see a growing number of travelers using them. They also come in handy when you are inside a rental car or an airport limousine service.

HOTEL ROOMS

You have just checked into your hotel room and are looking forward to a restful evening. Suddenly you smell toxic cleaning and laundry products, air fresheners, lingering perfume and/or cigarette smoke. What do you do?

▶ **Consider** *always* requesting a non-smoking room. If you do not receive one, ask to be moved to a smoke-free room. Depending on the extent to which you want to create an essential environment, here are several suggestions. Open all windows, if possible, to air out the room. It is sad, but even in the most polluted cities, the air outdoors has been found to be less toxic than the air indoors. Call housekeeping when you arrive and ask that they not use or spray any chemicals when cleaning your room. Pack your own chemical-free toiletries. Use a sleep sack, 100 percent cotton or silk sack that folds into a 3 x 5 inch, easy to pack, bundle. You can take your own 100 percent cotton pillowcase and towel to complete the package. Some hotels offer air purifiers using ionization and ozonation that you can request to be put inside your room to clear the air. It is best to leave the room while these units are running as they usually crank up the ozone output to clear the room faster than residential units. As ozone attaches to the particulate and renders it heavy enough to fall to the ground make sure housekeeping vacuums and dusts you room after the machine has been used.

NEW CAR INTERIORS
That wonderfully seductive aroma of a new car interior is *loaded* with toxins. Common materials such as plastic, vinyl, carpeting, and glue combine to release noxious fumes that can irritate eyes, nose and skin and can cause headaches and nausea. A Japanese research group found 114 harmful compounds in the fumes released in the interior of cars. Gas emissions from these chemicals have been linked to kidney and liver damage and other serious health problems. Softeners used in manufacturing plastic called phthalates are the most toxic offenders.

New car interiors have been found to be 45 times worse than the World Health Organization's standard for indoor air quality. Unsafe levels of emissions and volatile compounds are capable of remaining at a harmful level in the interior of a new car for months or even years.

▶ **Consider** keeping the windows open as much as possible for several months after buying a new car. Make sure the car has good ventilation and/or micro filters. A small bag of lava rocks or activated charcoal can be placed in the car to help remove most harmful gases and other pollutants. Obviously, purchasing cars in warm weather makes this an easier and more enjoyable task. You can also use a portable negative-ion generator in your car to neutralize the toxins. (See Sources.)

The International Center for Technology Assessment has established that the air inside moving cars is dirtier than the air outside of them. Pollutants enter from fumes emitted by the vehicle's engine. When following a diesel-driven vehicle, the pollutant level inside a car is six to eight times greater than if you were following a gasoline-fueled vehicle. Therefore, make sure your car is well ventilated when driving and that you avoid following diesel-fueled vehicles.

TAXI CABS, LIMOUSINES & RENTAL CARS

Give your taxi the "sniff and stay" or "sniff and no way" test. Hanging air fresheners, sprays and potpourri are usually toxic to breathe and they penetrate your skin, hair and clothing. Solutions that "cover-up" poor air quality are the cause of more chemical exposure and are best avoided.

▶ **Consider** asking for non-smoking and fragrance-free transportation. This is where making better choices truly makes a difference. When enough taxicab drivers get turned down because of toxic fragrances, they will stop using them.

Sometimes toxic fragrances cannot be avoided so use your personal negative-ion generating air purifier. You can also put a drop of your favorite essential oil on a tissue or handkerchief and hold it over your nose and mouth. Get out of the toxic zone as soon as possible.

Give your taxi the "sniff and stay" or "sniff and no way" test.

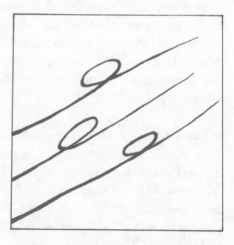

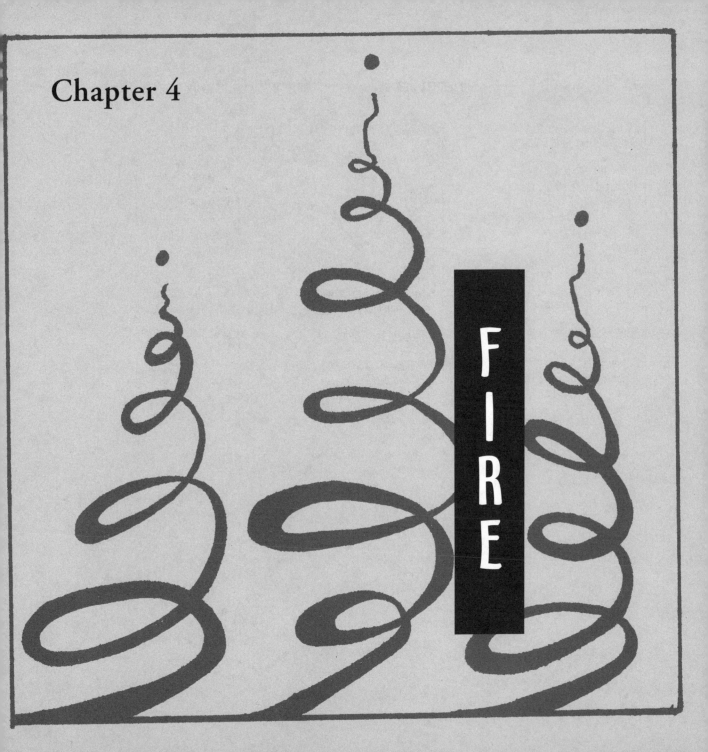

Chapter 4

FIRE

In This Chapter ⚞ Products and practices relating to food and drug choices

Introduction to Fire

Food, the fire that fuels the foundation of our life, is also the foundation for creating an essential environment within your body. Our food today has been so altered and processed that it has become quite unrecognizable fare. Instead of supplying us with energy and nutrition, our daily food intake only contributes to our consumption of preservatives, colorings, and additives, which in turn creates dis-ease, malnutrition, and ecological distress.

You do not have to look very far to see how sad our food supply has become. It is no coincidence that the acronym for the Standard American Diet is S.A.D! A multitude of information, as abundant as junk food itself, exists regarding what is wrong with our food industry. Although problems are much easier to write about than the solutions, I believe that you and I can navigate the path less taken and turn it into a path less toxic.

Our agricultural practices have created many complex issues surrounding our food supply. In response, we need to return vitality to our food by not supporting the companies and practices that promote these incredibly inferior foods of today. An overview of the problems underlying the S.A.D. will encourage us to move quickly onto the solutions. Becoming aware of these issues may lead you to eat toxic-free foods that are grown with sustainable agricultural practices. These suggestions will be of assistance as you begin to make better choices when purchasing, preparing and storing your food. After all, everything you do will be better when you fuel your body for health. It is possible, one simple step at a time.

Growing food has developed into big business—in the United States alone it is a $900 billion industry. Its policies are based on what is good for agribusiness and not on what is good for soil, animals and humans. The agricultural industry is disconnected from the flow of nature; it has a disrupting influence that affects everyone. Its guiding principle is focused on profits, not sustainable health—on greed, not nutrition. Our agricultural policies are determined by the agribusiness folks who, ironically, also just happen to be the largest political campaign contributors. Politics and profit will continue to go hand in hand with progress and pollution until we understand that our individual choices matter.

Common sense tells us that our agricultural policies and the dis-ease epidemic are connected yet there is not a single study linking agricultural subsidies to the status of our health. Our agricultural system is bottom line driven, not health driven. The incentive for agribusiness to create a safer food supply and support sustainable growing practices needs to come from you, the consumer. When we as global citizens embrace our individual power to become better consumers, the tide will change. Your choices coupled with all of our responsible choices will not be unnoticed.

Our diet has changed more in the last fifty years than it has in the previous fifty thousand years. This fifty-year experiment with our food has resulted in a serious diet-related, dis-ease epidemic. Agricultural practices have treated our resources and environment as being expendable and, in doing so, have compromised our health. Sad to say, we cannot trust that food *is* food anymore. Many of our food staples such as meat, fish and dairy products contain harmful chemicals, including traces of carcinogenic dioxins, additives, flavorings and colorings that our bodies do not know how to digest or eliminate. Today there is less and less food in our food.

The human body is a machine that is programmed to run on a certain kind of fuel. The proper fuel for the human body's peak performance is real, whole food—food that is free of chemicals, including pesticides, additives, flavorings, colorings, preservatives and sewage sludge fertilizer. When bodies are not properly fueled, they break down and exist in a state of dis-ease, not ease. We take better preventive care of our automobiles than we do of our bodies. We would never put water in our gas tanks and expect our cars to run, even though water would be less expensive and more convenient. Yet all day long we use cheaper and more convenient choices when fueling our bodies. Perhaps we need a sticker on our body to remind us when we need an "oil change," in this case, whole, organic food which represents a higher octane level of food in our tank instead of the lower grade regular fuel.

Digestion is the key to whole body health with weight loss as a fringe benefit. When your body can digest, process and eliminate the foods that you eat, it can be at ease, not dis-ease. Today's foods are mainly manufactured inside a factory with "value added substances" that the human body does not, and never will, recognize as food. At the turn of the century, the average grocery market had 50 food items on its shelves; today there are over 20,000, all made possible by chemicals that preserve food and extend shelf-life. Last year alone 28,000 new candies, ice cream and snack foods were introduced and only 230 fruit and vegetable products. Choosing to eat great tasting *and* nutritious foods that are easy-to-digest and chemical-free is the outline for an eating lifestyle that creates an essential environment in your body.

Cheap food is not always the most nutritious food. Farm subsidies were started during the Depression allowing farmers to make affordable food available. Government now

> *When your body can digest, process and eliminate the foods that you eat, it can be at ease, not dis-ease.*

spends billions of dollars annually on farm subsidizes in order to continue to provide inexpensive groceries to the consumer. Yet, regrettably, more inferior foods are subsidized than their nutritious counterparts. Less than 1 percent of the agricultural subsidies go to fruits and vegetables whereas refined sugars get twenty times that amount. Most of these subsidized farm products are used to make thousands of processed foods and livestock feed; in fact, 80 percent is the actual figure. Cheap and substandard ingredients in processed foods like sugar, water, salt, fat and artificial flavors have a higher profit margin. Organic food is priced right, other foods are cheap. Sometimes a bargain is not a bargain when the risk targets our health and well-being. Americans spend less of their discretionary income on food than any other nation in the world. Although quality food might be a bit more expensive at times, you are worth the investment.

Start by eating real, whole food. Know where your food comes from and who grows it. Ask what is in your food. Demand that food be put back into your food. Choose food that is free of chemicals, pesticides and toxic fertilizers. Read food labels. Buy food that is in season, because it greatly reduces the chances that it has been picked green or altered for storage. For example, apples are grown in the fall but chemicals and modern food processing enable them to be in grocery stores year round. Whenever possible, try to select locally grown food over artificially extended shelf life food. This choice supports the small farmer and cuts down on resources used to transport food. Discover the foods that are easiest to most difficult for your body to digest; as a result, your body does not have to work quite as hard while it heals.

You have great power as a consumer. You can begin to actually change what farmers grow by exercising your consumer power. Purchase quality, organic foods and return to the salvation, not starvation, of your kitchen. Avoid cheap food ingredients, such as refined white flour, refined white sugar, white rice and foods that contain chemical flavorings and additives. Demand quality, honest labeling, and safety from your food sources and suppliers.

Considerations for Fire

On a regular basis give yourself a pep talk just to make sure convenience foods and food marketers do not lull you back into a state of delusion that keeps you from taking the next simple step toward good health. After all, everything you do, from playing with your children to a job interview, is subsequently enhanced when you live in a healthy body. Put your dollars where they will make a difference in your world. Your food choices matter.

This chapter on food is divided into 6 categories: Buy, Cook & Store Chemical-free Foods; Food Alterations; Food Processing; Food Related Dis-ease; Food Related Topics and Specific Foods. Each topic will assist you in fueling your body for better health and better living. Take one page at a time and realize that you are worth it.

Buy, Cook & Store Chemical-Free Food

COOKING

Cooking, an activity that had fallen out of vogue, is returning to our culture as an activity that is social, sensual, simple and smart. Cooking is the core of our existence and can raise the energy level in an environment. It is a great activity that unites families, friends and neighbors. Today, we have more cooking equipment and gadgets, more space to cook in, yet we spend less time preparing food than any other culture since the beginning of time. To heal your body, toxic foods need to be removed from your diet. Cooking your own food is a great way to begin.

Cooking once or twice a week provides you with the prepared ingredients for putting meals together in minutes.

▶ **Consider** that not everyone *has* the time to cook from scratch. Realizing this, I developed the concept of the Continuous Kitchen. Cooking once or twice a week provides you with the prepared ingredients for putting meals together in minutes. Roast a tray of vegetables, bake a chicken, cook a pan of cornbread, and make a treat. *Essential Eating, A Cookbook: Discover How To Eat, Not Diet* has 350 easy recipes to get you started, including shopping lists, menus and sample Continuous Kitchen cooking sessions. Cooking is a wonderful activity for all, men, women, and children. If you seek a healthier you, cooking will serve you well.

If you want to restore your health, build better relationships, slow your life down or get in touch with yourself, bring a little cooking back into your life.

Try this easy and delicious snack to get a little cooking back into your life. It takes all of 4 minutes.

Edamame	*(Fresh Soy Beans)*
	1 bag frozen organic edamame in the pods

Place a steamer pot on the stove, add about ½ inch of water to cover bottom; bring to a boil. Add edamame, cover and steam for 4 minutes. Remove from stove and run cold water over to cool. Sprinkle with a touch of salt and eat. Use your fingers to break open the side of the pod and eat the fresh bean inside. Because this wonderful snack is packaged in its own shell, it is easy to transport.

COOKWARE, UTENSILS & CUTTING BOARDS

Yikes! Recent media has led us to ask questions about the safety of non-stick cookware. Some reports state that when non-stick cookware heats to high temperatures, ultra-fine particles break off and can become imbedded in your lungs, causing flu-like symptoms that can last for a few days. Lawsuits concerning chemical exposure are pending involving women who attribute the chemicals applied to non-stick cookware to their babies' birth defects. A recent report stated that some parakeets are now being sold with instructions that state, "Please do not put the bird in the kitchen where fumes from non-stick cookware could be harmful or even fatal."

▶ **Consider** getting the non-stick cookware out of your life. Why wait for the government or even less likely, cookware companies, to tell us that the non-stick coating is toxic? Just use pots and pans that are safe, stainless steel, glass, cast iron, enameled cast iron, ceramic and stoneware. No explanations needed. Again, this is a situation where your consumer buying power *can* impact an industry.

Use stainless steel utensils instead of plastic for cooking and dining. Wooden spoons and silver are fine.

Wood or bamboo cutting boards are durable and come from a sustainable source. Marble or granite can also be used, but it is a bit heavy and will dull your knives faster. If possible, have two cutting boards, one for meat and the other for everything else. Always wash thoroughly with soap and warm water.

FARMERS & THEIR MARKETS

The number of American farmers has plummeted by 300,000 since 1979. This trend will continue as agribusiness farms grow larger and more centralized. There are currently 2 million farms in America with 94 percent being small farms run primarily by families. The movement toward a few, centralized, large, vertically integrated farms controlling the majority of food and fiber products only benefits large agribusiness companies.

Ten companies supply more than half the food and drink sold in the United States. It is not a matter of volume since we grow twice as much food as we consume; it is a matter of quality.

Although big agribusiness experts are in favor of this centralizing trend as a way to provide efficient food products, they have not taken into consideration the destruction to the environment caused by large livestock operations, chemically-laden soil and perhaps more importantly, the loss of competition. It is a myth that organic farmers produce a lower yield than conventional farmers. Since the quality of the soil determines production, organic farmers will be exceeding conventional farmers for years to come. In fact, most of the larger operating farms use more energy through chemical fertilizing. Combine that with the energy required to process the food, and the transportation fuel required, the finished product has demanded more energy to produce than the food itself can calorically provide.

During the Colonial Period in our nation's history, it was observed that Americans were at least a head taller than their British counterparts. This was attributed to the fact that the American soil was not as depleted as the British soil. The Colonists were planting in a rich, thick, and abundant blanket of topsoil and the benefits were apparent in the health of the people who ate the crops. Today, the depletion of valuable nutrients that are inherent in top soil, ironically, is also evident in the health of Americans.

> *The Colonists were planting in a rich, thick, and abundant blanket of topsoil and the benefits were apparent in the health of the people who ate the crops.*

▶ **Consider** that by not buying cheap, processed foods you will support the small farmer. Whenever possible, buy locally grown foods and products at your farmers market. Be sure to ask questions because all of the foods sold at farmers markets are not always grown by local farmers or free of pesticides. Small farmers are usually willing to discuss what methods they use in growing their products. Ask questions and then you can decide.

For everyone to be able to eat a healthy diet, twice as many fruits and vegetables would have to be planted. Buying a variety of fruits and vegetables will support diversity among our food growers. Diversity of crops is also a healthy scenario for the soil because the likelihood of nutrient depletion lessens.

U-pick farms and roadside farm stands are also a good way to buy fresh, flavorful produce and, at the same time, support your local producer. To support their local organic farmers, some communities are establishing buying clubs to increase demand for local produce. Many farmers deliver produce directly to consumers.

Support the organic revolution by demanding to know what you are eating and how it was grown. Buying organic food preserves our soil, protects our water and supports the small farmer. The American agricultural system will only be transformed by your buying power.

GARDENS

Agriculture is being consolidated into a shrinking number of corporate hands. This is not a good thing.

▶ **Consider** in addition to supporting small farmers, you could plant a garden. Even a garden in a small planter on your patio will lend a hand. You might join Community Supported Agriculture (CSA). You can buy CSA shares with the produce serving as your dividend. Often times they give you the option of working to reduce the cost of your share. Another option is joining a food cooperative which is usually known for supporting the locally grown producers and is a source for safe foods. (See Farmers & Their Markets.)

If planting a garden is out of the question, then be sure to choose organic, chemical-free, unadulterated, GMO-free foods when possible. This will eventually send a message to corporate farming that we want real food that is not based on perfection or price.

GRILLING

When meat is grilled over high heat, the fat drips onto the heat source (coals, wood, gas flames and electric coils). This, in turn, causes potentially cancer-causing chemicals to be absorbed by the food from the rising smoke; and as a result, heterocyclic amines (HCAs) are formed. High intake levels of HCAs are linked to an increased risk of pancreatic, colorectal and stomach cancers.

▶ **Consider** that if you cannot live without grilling, reduce your risk to these hazardous chemicals by using low-fat cuts of meat and trimming all visible fat. Push the coals to the sides of the grill once they are hot so meat is not directly above them. Protect meat from the smoke by either wrapping it in foil or placing a baking sheet between the meat and the coals to catch the fat drippings.

Cooking the meat on medium or low heat will drastically cut HCA formation when grilling. Remove meat before it is well-done as longer cooking times increase HCAs. Cut off any charred bits from the meat.

PURCHASING FOOD

We are great consumers, that is, until it comes to buying food. When we buy material possessions like a car or a television we are determined to know everything about it. We automatically equate higher price with better quality. Yet, when faced with a decision between food priced at .99 and $1.29, most customers pick the lower priced item—hands down with no questions asked. We are dreadful food consumers.

▶ **Consider** that just like other material possessions, the higher the price of food the better the quality. Real, organic food may cost a few cents more at times, but the benefits your body derives from it are priceless. In the long run, buying real, organic food is cheaper, considering the cost of drugs to fight indigestion and dis-ease. Buying good food supports your health and the farmers who are committed to growing real food in a way that preserves and sustains our precious earth. You can become a better food consumer. Buy fresh food that is unprocessed and chemical-free. Do not be held hostage by convenience foods that are robbing you of your health.

STORING FOOD

Bacteria can easily grow in and on food if it has not been handled and stored properly. Foods left out of the refrigerator are more likely to be candidates for bacteria growth.

▶ **Consider** storing your food in glass, stainless steel, ceramic, or waxed paper. These materials are all toxin-free and therefore will not add chemicals to your food. Keep refrigerated foods in the refrigerator as much as possible. Frozen foods should be thawed in the refrigerator or in cold water. Reheat foods to at least 165 degrees to assure harmful microorganisms are destroyed. Always wash hands thoroughly before and after handling food. Be sure to wash any equipment that has come into contact with food.

N.E.E.D.S., Nutritional, Ecological, Environmental Delivery System is a mail order company that sells two sizes of cellophane bags, made from wood pulp. They are a wonderful, sustainable, reusable, compostable alternative to plastic bags. (See Sources.)

TRANSPORTATION OF FOOD

With the consolidation of food growers, food is being transported for longer distances. This creates a push for longer shelf life through chemical additives and genetic modification.

Buying good food supports your health and the farmers who are committed to growing real food in a way that preserves and sustains our precious earth.

▶ **Consider** buying food and products that are grown locally when possible. Not only will this save on transportation resources, but the food is likely to be fresher and more nutritious. Grocery shop once or twice a week to cut down on your personal transportation of food and to check out the fresh arrivals.

Food Alterations

ADDITIVES

Food additives include preservatives, colorings, flavorings, sweeteners and any novel substance that is added to food. By law, any novel substance added to a food must, unless it is "generally recognized as safe" (GRAS), be thoroughly tested. If the substance alters the product in any manner, it must be listed on the label.

Unfortunately, many of the chemicals that make up product flavorings are not required to be disclosed seeing that they are considered GRAS. "Generally" is the wiggle word here. Almost all processed foods necessitate flavor additives. Artificial and natural flavorings sometimes contain the same volatile chemicals, but are a result of different production methods. Both artificial and natural flavorings are made from chemicals; however, it is the method of extraction that creates the difference in the end result.

Today food manufacturers use a chemical called glutamate as a taste enhancer. The most familiar form of glutamate is known to consumers as monosodium glutamate (MSG). A vast amount of controversy surrounds the health risks of MSG. Some people have linked MSG to migraine headaches, skin rashes, Autism, Attention Deficit Disorder and severe depression. Pregnant women, infants and the health conscious are warned not to consume foods containing MSG. MSG is reported by some to have addictive effects and that food manufacturers use it to make people eat more. The real debate should be over the actual labeling not the ingredient itself. Although labeled as a chemical, MSG can also be a hidden component in other ingredients. Unknowingly, we often purchase foods that we think are free of MSG.

The confusion is fueled by the use of other ingredients that contain significant levels of glutamate such as potassium glutamate, hydrolyzed vegetable protein, plant protein extract, yeast extract, textured protein, sodium caseinate and others that are unknown to most consumers. MSG can also be included as a smaller percentage of other additives to avoid label requirements.

The FDA is not fulfilling its pledge to consumers when it provides inadequate labeling guidelines for manufacturers to abide by and then leaves the consumer questioning product ingredients. If MSG is capable of being a stowaway ingredient, we will all finally end up paying for its fare by suffering ill health. If it is so safe, why do they work so hard to conceal MSG and other chemicals in our food that may place humans at risk? Because they know we are capable of being smart shoppers and intelligent voters!

Millions of tons of MSG and other glutamates are also used routinely in many soaps, salad dressings, canned tuna fish, vegetables and soups, frozen food entrees, low-fat processed foods, ice cream, processed meats, baby food and even some vaccines. Until MSG is properly labeled, avoiding these food items. Even some foods that are labeled "No MSG" have been found to contain traces of MSG. Watch for key words such as seasonings and flavorings which, more often than not, contain MSG. Again, know that you are capable of taking responsibility for your health by making better selections.

Aspartame is another food additive surrounded by controversy. Aspartame is a chemical used to replace the sugar in sugar-free foods like gum and diet soft drinks. As with so many other debates, until this one is settled, why take the risk? Why use this artificial sweetener when you can consume an alternative that will support your health without question? Instead, try granulated maple sugar—a whole food, not a chemical.

Another ingredient being added to processed foods as a sweetener and bulking agent is sugar alcohol. Do not be confused, it is neither sugar nor alcohol. Sugar alcohol is often added to "sugar-free" food products such as cookies, soft drinks, candies and chewing gums to give them a sweet flavor. Read the labels—common sugar alcohols are mannitol, sorbitol, xylitol, lactitol, isomalt, maltitol and hydrogenated starch hydrolysates (HSH). The positive side of sugar alcohols is that they contain fewer calories than sugar, and they do not promote tooth decay. The negative side is that actual weight gain has been experienced when sugar alcohols are overeaten. Due to the way these chemicals digest, they can cause diarrhea and bloating when consumed in excessive amounts.

Foods containing additives are easy to find. Think about the places you obtain food in the course of your day—a convenient store, vending machine, sporting event, hospital, school, food court, a fast food outlet or movie theatre. *None* of these outlets offer *real food* that is free of additives.

▶ **Consider** that more and more of us are realizing that fake foods are making us sick and considerably overweight. Cultural changes will occur when more of us stop buying junk

Instead of purchasing processed sugary snacks that are filled with additives, take along some pure maple candies.

food that is filled with chemicals. By introducing a little cooking into your daily life you will be able to eat real, chemical-free foods that support your health.

When you are away from home, instead of purchasing processed sugary snacks that are filled with additives, take along some pure maple candies. They are made from one hundred percent maple syrup which is the easiest to digest sweetener. Maple products are a whole food. You can eat the maple candy or dissolve it in a cup of herbal tea. It is a delicious treat without preservatives or additives.

DIOXINS

Dioxins are considered the most poisonous man-made, organic chemical. It affects the human endocrine system by disrupting the human hormone function including the thyroid gland, adrenal and reproductive systems.

Dioxins accumulate in our soil, water and in the fatty tissues of animals and humans. They are also released into the air through the burning of trash. In some fast food and grocery store staples, studies show them at levels that exceed US government standards by 200 percent or more.

Exposure can cause cancer, heart disease, infertility, and diabetes. The younger the exposure to dioxin, the more dis-ease it causes. Children can be exposed to dioxin during the prenatal stage, causing developmental problems.

▶ **Consider** eating fewer animal products since 90 percent of our personal exposure to dioxin comes through meat and dairy products. Make sure your meat and dairy products are low-fat and come from organically fed animals.

Consume local products whenever possible. Globalization means foods may be produced under conditions that are not safe, allowing the use of dioxin-contaminated pesticides on produce. Purchasing local products tremendously cuts down on the uncertainty of your food sources and the growing, storing, and marketing practices.

Buy foods that are not wrapped in plastic when possible. Wash all fruits and vegetables thoroughly. Peel waxed produce.

GENETICALLY MODIFIED FOODS

The science behind genetically modified (GM) food or organisms is called food biotechnology—the use of modern genetics to alter plants, animals and microorganisms. In 1998, forty-five million acres of American farmland was planted with GM, sometimes called genetically engineered or biotech crops. These GM crops consisted mostly of corn, soybeans, cotton and potatoes. The transfer of genes between completely unrelated organisms allows for GM crops to perform unlike they would naturally such as producing their own pesticides, withstanding herbicides and extending shelf-life. Unlike GM crops, traditional farming techniques use natural processes to bring about changes in foods, not processes that allow combinations of species unlikely to occur naturally. Our food chain stands in need of reform, but biological and chemical alteration is not the answer. We need to naturally replenish our soil and ecologically strengthen our crops. Agricultural technology needs to be sustainable, which it is not at the present time.

We have such a poor understanding of how an organism develops that we are quite possibly in for a rude awakening as biotech crops infiltrate our environment. There are no safe-guard tests to determine if biotech crops will produce super weeds and resistant insects. Genetically modified organisms (GMO) do not support an essential environment because their consequences are unpredictable and usually requires more counter action or deterrence which once again introduces more toxins and more ramifications. We are so entangled in the administering of chemicals that we are now seeing the effects of the chemical offspring of their forefathers such as DDT (dichlorodiphenyltrichloroethane), a banned pesticide.

Genetically modified organisms (GMO) do not support an essential environment because their consequences are unpredictable.

Until food companies are capable of assuring us that genetically modified, altered or engineered foods are safe and will not cross pollinate (seems impossible) with organic crops and eventually contaminate our entire food supply, buy and eat GMO-free foods. We have no idea of the long-term effects of GMO foods on humans or our ecosystem. Always check the food labels to see that the food product is GMO-free or organic.

In Europe, where genetically engineered food is required to be labeled, consumers choose to buy GMO-free foods over the labeled GMO foods. In response to this measure, the United States politicians actually passed a law stating that GMO foods do not need to be labeled! Trust your own judgment on this one; buy and eat GMO-free foods.

Although 94 percent of Americans want GMO foods to be labeled, 74 percent of them are not aware when and if they have eaten GMO foods. Not such a surprising statistic when 80 percent of the foods sitting on the United States grocery store shelves contain genetically modified foods that are not labeled. A reverse labeling has occurred in that companies not using GMO foods are now labeling them GMO-free.

The following is an example of how GMO foods can jeopardize your health. One of my friends is allergic to nuts. One day while eating lunch, she had to be rushed to the hospital due to an attack of epileptic shock. The doctor was perplexed since nothing in her lunch appeared to contain nuts. Months later she was reading an article about a group of growers who had genetically crossed a tomato with a Brazil nut attempting to make it more pest-resistant and to create a longer shelf life. This was the culprit that sent her to the hospital. She did not know the tomato contained organisms from a Brazil nut. Who would have? Consumers beware; buy and eat GMO-free foods.

▶ **Consider** the fact that when you buy certified organic foods, they do not contain GMOs. Buying organic food sends a message to biotech growers that you are not interested in their food.

Biological and chemical pollution will be the environmental challenge of the future. We can all take that one simple step today by not buying these foods. You can do it. We all can do it. It will make a difference, a positive difference!

IRRADIATED FOODS

Irradiating food is the equivalent of exposing it up to 1 billion chest x-rays. Foods such as beef, chicken, turkey, vegetables, fruit, eggs, pork, juice and sprouted seeds can be legally irradiated to reduce bacteria and extend shelf life. Although irradiation does kill certain harmful microorganisms, it does not remove the feces, urine and other animal fluids often inherent in modern food processing.

There are experts on both sides stating their arguments for and against irradiated foods. Since being introduced in 1999, it has not been received with consumer confidence. When introduced in Europe, irradiated foods were labeled and the consumers' preference for non-irradiated foods was obvious. In America, irradiated food is not required to be labeled making it harder for the consumer to make a choice. Some conscientious companies are now labeling their foods non-irradiated.

Irradiated foods were not permitted in public school meal programs until recently. Although each school system has the choice, the Los Angeles School System voted not to use irradiated foods in their meal programs. Good job.

▶ **Consider** that the discussion ought to be about how to grow and to process food that does not need to be irradiated. Until that happens, you need to ask these questions:

Where is this food grown? How is it processed? What, if any, chemicals are used? Is it irradiated? Again, find safe sources for your food and get to know your food suppliers.

The jury is still out as to whether irradiated food is safe for human consumption. That is all I need to know. Case closed!

LABELING

By the time you cut through all of the legislation related to food labeling, it is safe to say it is not always reliable. Safe food labeling is determined by the agendas of politicians, agribusiness, scientists, chemical producers, the Federal Food and Drug Administration, the United States Department of Agriculture, the Environmental Protection Agency (EPA)– the list goes on. An entire work could be devoted to this subject alone. I will just mention a few simple concepts that will help you make better buying decisions when reading food labels. Right now, our reactions as consumers is the best form of reform that we can offer. We have to convince big business that they can no longer just do what is most convenient and then repent!

Cage-free, free-range and free-roaming.

If all animals were treated humanely, these phrases would not be necessary.

The real money in agriculture is the 90 percent value added to the food we eat. These figures are calculated and controlled by selling what is called inputs, the chemicals, fertilizers and pesticides sold to the farmers, and then processing their crops. Most farmers are undergoing a sense of guilt about using chemicals to grow food. However, because of economics, they are forced to use chemicals or go out of business. Unfortunately, pesticides and many of the added chemicals in food are not required to be listed on food labels.

If you do not know what an ingredient is, chances are it is a chemical additive and you should avoid it. Other foods to steer clear of include those containing tropical oils, hydrogenated oils, refined foods, artificial *and* natural flavorings, colorings, and additives. Trans fats should be avoided at all costs or profits.

A few phrases that have burst onto the food labeling scene are "cage-free", "free-range" and "free-roaming." If all animals were treated humanely, these phrases would not be necessary. Reports on of the food industry's inhumane housing of animals has caused consumers be sympathetic to these phrases. These phrases on food labels are open to a wide range of interpretation, but they cannot be interpreted as organic. The USDA's National Organic Program (N.O.P) states that whether or not an animal has been caged does not determine what types of feed they were given.

Products labeled "natural" or "all natural" are not the same as organic. The USDA's

N.O.P neither defines nor regulates the use of these words. Although products labeled "natural" may not include added colorings or flavorings, it does not mean that the product was derived through organic means. "Natural" products can also be "minimally processed." Keep in mind that the words "healthy" and "lite" on food labels do not necessarily mean that they will support your health.

►**Consider** that the time you spend reading the ingredients on food labels is time well spent.

When reading labels, support companies that treat animals and our earth humanely. The phrases, "100 percent organic," "organic" or "made with organic" are the only phrases sanctioned by the USDA's N.O.P to assure a food product is organic. Organic, sustainable farming goes to great lengths to preserve the whole ecosystem, including animal and human health.

PACKAGING

Upon becoming acquainted with the negative impact of plastic, you will probably question, and rightly so, why so much of our food is packaged and stored in plastic. Food packaging using poly vinyl chloride (PVC) can include plastic trays in boxed cookies or crackers, candy bar wrappers, and bottles. Plastic cling wraps, especially the kind used commercially to wrap cheeses, produce, meats and other foods, can also be comprised of PVC. Unfortunately, many people are exposed to plasticizing chemicals through food wrapping every day. Again, it comes down to economics. Although plastic is extremely toxic to both humans and our environment, it is less costly for food manufacturers. Of course the cost of your health, my health, and the earth's integrity is not considered due to the economics of using plastic.

►**Consider** that you have a choice. You can opt for food that is packaged and stored in glass, cellophane, stainless steel, paper or waxed paper. Even better, select food products that are not pre-packaged. If the food you buy is wrapped in plastic, transfer it to a glass or stainless steel container at home. Storing your food in glass or stainless steel containers, cellophane or waxed paper prevents the toxicity from being absorbed from the packing material.

Fortunately, many companies are seeking earth-friendly packaging solutions. One in particular, Wild Oats Natural Marketplace, is selling food in containers made from a familiar yet renewable resource, corn. Containers that are returned to the store are delivered to a local composting facility where they will decompose within forty to fifty days. This compost is then used as an all natural plant food. Good job! Great consideration!

PESTICIDES

Farmers annually apply almost 600 million pounds of pesticides, including herbicides, fungicides and insecticides that invariably end up contaminating our ground water and infiltrating our food, animals, plants, and air. Many of these pesticides, categorized as carcinogenic by the EPA, are considered to cause cancer, heart disease, genetic damage, immune disorders, kidney and liver damage, among a host of other health problems. These harmful chemicals can penetrate our bodies through the foods that we eat.

Atrazine, America's most widely used pesticide, used primarily for killing insects or for insect control, has been linked to cancer in humans. It has been banned in Europe. The debate about which pesticides are safe will continue. Some argue that the EPA is being too cautious, but what can be considered too cautious when it comes to your health?

Remember, all pesticides are toxic to something. The Environmental Protection Agency has established human "tolerances" for each chemical and then subjects it to a risk-benefit analysis. What has not been taken into consideration with this "single chemical" analysis is the human risk suffered from exposure to the intense *combination* of all pesticides from many different sources and as many differing levels of toxicity. A dangerous chemical cannot be adequately assessed nor can its inherent harm be appropriately addressed when monitored in such a vacuum type testing area. The interactions of the various strains of toxic chemicals in our environment create their own reactions. The damage is usually already done invalidating the EPAs single chemical test results.

▶ **Consider** buying organic foods which help protect you from harmful chemicals. Thoroughly wash fruits and vegetables and peel waxed produce. Buy whole foods versus processed foods.

Use your buying power to change your world. Preventing the use of pesticides might be a bigger challenge that any individual wants to contemplate. So for now, buy foods and products that do not use pesticides.

Use your buying power to change your world.

PRESERVATIVES

Originally, preservatives were created to provide food safety, rapid transit and ideal storage conditions. Unfortunately, the chemicals used to preserve foods have not always proven safe.

The list of side effects from preservatives is endless and the use of these chemicals has escalated in an attempt to increase the shelf life of food. Commercially-prepared foods have transformed chemical additives into a significantly major part of our diet. Many of these chemicals are poorly tested and always pose the threat of being potentially dangerous, especially foods that contain sodium nitrate, saccharin, caffeine, acesulfame K and artificial colorings.

▶ **Consider** avoiding foods that contain preservatives. A great rule to follow is do not buy or eat anything with ingredients that you cannot pronounce or that contain unfamiliar ingredients. A great book called *Food Additives*, by Ruth Winter, M.S., is a virtual encyclopedia describing in plain English more that 8,000 food additives.

Food Processing

AIRLINE FOOD

Just say, "No, thank you." Recently, while engaged in a conversation with a flight attendant about my book, *Essential Eating*, she laughed and replied "You certainly do not want to eat airline food; it is the farthest thing from being organic. It is sprayed with preservatives to make it look good for a long time, even if it has to be reheated multiple times."

Airline food service companies encounter great challenges in their attempt to serve food to passengers. Take into account the processing food goes through and the number of people handling it from harvesting to packaging. It certainly is not fresh nor is it free of preservatives. In fact, most of the airline food is encrusted with preservatives and is loaded with additives to make it look appealing for a long period of time. To add insult to injury, much of the airline food is also microwaved on plastic plates.

▶ **Consider** taking your own brown bag on board. Even a picnic box from a hotel is a far better choice than airline food. In an effort to cut costs, it may be a blessing that airlines are discontinuing their in-flight meal service. Do yourself a big favor and pack a sandwich. Try an ALT—avocado, lettuce and tomato sandwich.

ALT Sandwich	(serves 2)
	4 slices of *sprouted* grain bread
	1 ripe avocado
	1 small tomato
	2 large lettuce leaves
	2 tablespoons yogurt cheese or cream cheese

Toast the bread, peel and thinly slice the avocado. Wash tomato and lettuce, slice tomato. Spread one tablespoon yogurt cheese on each of the two slices of bread. Divide avocado, tomato and lettuce and layer over yogurt cheese. Top with remaining slices of bread.

Note: Yogurt cheese is made by straining the whey out of yogurt. Place plain yogurt in cheesecloth suspended over a bowl for 4 hours or overnight.

Also, avoid caffeinated and alcoholic beverages in flight since they act as a diuretic and can cause dehydration and headaches. Spring water or juice is a better choice.

FAST FOOD

The fast-food industry has been receiving a great deal of distressing press lately. Fast food is not whole food; it never was and never will be! A cheeseburger from a major fast-food chain has been sitting on a plate in my office for the past *three* years. It also travels around the country with me and is famous for being on television. The remarkable thing is that it has not changed in three years—no rot, no mold, and no decay. It is a classic example of how chemicals preserve food. If this burger cannot be broken down in three years sitting on my desk, how can your body adequately process and eliminate it? If you believe that you get what you pay for, do not expect a meal bought for a dollar or two to be capable of nurturing your health.

One can only surmise that the "Personal Responsibility in Food Consumption Act" is being pushed through Congress is a result of recent lawsuits from consumers stating that fast-food made them fat. This Act, also known as the "Cheeseburger Bill", bans people from suing food manufacturers, sellers and distributors; even if it is proven that they added harmful chemicals to their food products. The food industry lobbyists do not want to follow in the footsteps of the tobacco industry that was exposed when consumers demanded payment for the harmful effects of Nicotine.

Every day and everywhere chain restaurants are being built. Do not be fooled. These chain restaurants are just fancy fast-food outlets. Their adorned concrete block structures offer food that is processed and packaged elsewhere. There is not a chef in the kitchen peeling potatoes—it is usually a boil-in-a-bag cuisine with food being assembled, not prepared.

We spend more money annually on fast food than on new cars, higher education, and personal computers. One generation ago 75 percent of our food budgets were allocated to purchasing food in order to prepare meals at home. Today, almost 50 percent of our food budget is spent at restaurants. It is also reported that 50 percent more calories, fat and sodium are consumed when eating out.

▶ **Consider** getting a little cooking back into your active life. You will then have a better idea of what is in your food and how it is prepared. It is really much easier than you think. It will not only simplify your life but also restore your health. With a little planning, you can cook once or twice a week and have ingredients ready to put meals together in minutes.

Even the salads at fast-food outlets are not healthy. The largest part of these salads consists mainly of iceberg lettuce which has zero nutrients and zero grams of fiber. Still, the average American eats twenty-five pounds of iceberg lettuce annually. The accompanying salad dressings made available to the consumer sometimes contain more grams of fat than the burgers from the same establishment. Make and pack your own salad with nutritious lettuce such as romaine, spinach, arugula or mixed greens, topped with sprouts and vegetables and dressed with an olive oil and vinegar based dressing. Or instead of going out for fast-food, stay home and try this easy and delicious recipe.

Oven Fried Chicken	*(serves 8)*
	6 slices sprouted bread
	1½ tablespoons fresh thyme leaves, (or 1¼ teaspoons dried)
	1½ tablespoons fresh rosemary, (or 1¼ teaspoons dried)
	1 teaspoon salt
	1 teaspoon pepper
	3 cups plain yogurt
	4 pounds chicken pieces

Toast bread until crisp. Cool. Tear into chunks and place in food processor. Pulse until bread turns into crumbs. Add thyme and rosemary and pulse until finely chopped. Pour crumbs into a bowl, add salt and pepper. Put yogurt in a separate bowl. Preheat oven to 400 degrees. Clean chicken, dip in yogurt and then roll in seasoned crumbs. Arrange chicken pieces on a large greased baking sheet and bake 45 minutes, or until golden brown and cooked throughout. Serve hot or at room temperature.

KOSHER FOOD

Many certified organic products also carry the kosher label. Kosher is the Hebrew word for fit or proper. Kosher food laws were established in Biblical times to prohibit the contamination of one food type by another. Although this ancient food-safety practice continues today, it does not guarantee that kosher food is safer or any purer unless it is labeled organic.

▶ **Consider** that for those of us who are concerned about increased pollutants in our food, most kosher food producers promote the purity of foods by avoiding hormones, antibiotics or artificial flavorings. Get to know your food suppliers and ask questions about how your food is grown and what practices are used in its processing.

MICROWAVED FOOD

We could not locate one study published by the small appliance industry on the effects of microwaving on the human body. Quite possibly a study has been compiled but is not being released. Do not wait.

Instead, think of microwaved meals as food that has run a marathon in seconds. How does a body feel after running a marathon—tired, breathless, spent? Microwaved food does not seem to provide the same energy, taste or consistency of food that has been prepared conventionally. The intensity of microwaved food completely cancels out the healing concept of eating fresh, quality food that is as close to its original state as possible.

▶ **Consider** that with just a little advanced planning, conventional cooking can be almost as fast. From the freezer to the microwave to the table is not the path to feeling good. Your safest choice is still fresh, quality food which has been cooked conventionally. For

Your safest choice is still fresh, quality food which has been cooked conventionally.

example, an organic baked potato cooked conventionally and topped with butter is a better choice than frozen fried potatoes that have been "nuked."

ORGANIC FOOD

Food did not require organic labeling before chemicals were introduced into our agriculture practices. Our food was grown organically prior to the chemical revolution. In October 2002, National Organic Standards went into effect, requiring that all food products labeled as organic must meet stringent standards established by the US Department of Agriculture (USDA). Organic refers to the way food, animals, and fibers are grown and processed. It supports an ecological system that relies on healthy, rich soil to produce strong plants that resist pests and diseases. Organic farming prohibits the use of toxic chemicals in favor of earth- and human-friendly practices that work in harmony with nature. Genetically modified organisms (GMOs) and antibiotics are prohibited in organic farming.

Organic products fall into one of three USDA labeling categories. The first label is 100 percent organic—made with 100 percent organic ingredients. The second label is organic—made with at least 95 percent organic ingredients, with strict restrictions on the remaining 5 percent of the ingredients, including no GMOs. The third label states made with organic ingredients—made with a minimum of 70 percent organic ingredients with strict restrictions on the remaining 30 percent including no GMOs.

▶ **Consider** that organic practices heal you and repair our world. Unlike conventional farming, organic farming does not contaminate the soil, infect farm workers or infest our food supply. Likewise, chemicals do not run off and contaminate our water supply. Organic practices support a sustainable environment which in turn supports you.

Due to the increased consumer demand for organic foods, organic junk foods are finding their way onto grocery store shelves. Even though consumers now have organic labeling laws on their side, be attentive to the fact that all food labeled organic is not guaranteed to be good for your health. Choose organic whole foods such as produce, grains, nuts, eggs and meats. Stay away from organic junk foods including organic donuts, pastries and processed foods. They simply represent another lesson in denial. By being honest with yourself, both your health and weight goals will be easier to attain.

When you have a choice, buy organic. Organic foods are the *only* foods that prohibit the use of genetically engineered organisms, irradiation, sewage sludge and cloned animals.

When you are unable to find organic foods, due to temporary circumstances, use the following list to help you make acceptable and smart substitutes. Some of the foods that are the most contaminated by pesticides and chemicals are apples, peppers, celery, cherries, potatoes, eggs, meats, strawberries, red raspberries, imported grapes, imported cantaloupe, cucumbers, peaches, pears and spinach. The foods with the least amount of contamination include asparagus, avocados, bananas, broccoli, cauliflower, coconuts, kiwis, mangoes, onions, papayas, pineapples and sweet peas.

If you are concerned about the increased cost of organic produce, factor in the cost of your doctor bills, increased insurance premiums and prescription medicine. Organic foods will always come out less expensive. Think of organic food as your investment for healthy living.

Share the benefits of eating real food with a young person today. They do eventually learn what they live.

PROCESSED FOOD

Ninety percent of new and improved foods are packaged junk foods. The food industry has become very smart and very profitable. What incentives are provided to induce companies to sacrifice profits for improved public health?—to this point none.

▶ **Consider**, optimistically, we will become the incentive, hidden under the guise of lost sales and the consumer's powerfully voiced discontent. When the registers stop ringing, the silence will be overwhelming and the consumer perhaps will play a larger and more effective part in what the food market decides to dish out.

SLOW FOOD

The Slow Food movement started in Italy when an activist, Carlo Petrini, decided to counteract fast food using a long-term strategy intended to rescue food from homogenization. Slow Food calls for environmental awareness, sustainable agriculture and the education of young children on the pitfalls of mass-produced and fast food. It promotes the cultivation of foods in customs that support our environment and preserve indigenous crops. Slow Food followers exist in forty-five countries and include seventy thousand members.

► **Consider** that you can join the Slow Food movement by becoming aware of the simple practice of being an improved food consumer. We have seen the unhealthy benefits of fast food, why not try slow food. Share the benefits of eating real food with a young person today. They do eventually learn what they live. The important thing is that we become the example as advocates of real food.

Food Related Dis-ease

CHEWING

Our ancestors certainly had a valid point behind their preaching to "chew your food more." Our express lives do not allow much time for eating, let alone dining or mindful chewing. Because digestion begins in the mouth, chewing creates saliva that sets in motion the process of breaking down the cell walls of food.

► **Consider** that by chewing each bite of food thoroughly, you will have better digestion, as well as elimination. Taking time to savor and experience each mouthful will remove unnecessary stress from the digestive system while supplying a pleasant taste sensation as a bonus.

CRAVINGS

Certain foods, such as chocolates, cheeses, sugars, meats and starches, stimulate the same part of the brain as alcohol, heroin and tobacco. These foods release a feel-good chemical in the brain called dopamine. These good feelings inadvertently lead to cravings that in turn can lead to overeating and addiction.

Chocolate contains many substances, including stimulants, such as theobromine and phenylethylamine and a small amount of anandamide. Combine these substances with the caffeine in chocolate and your body gets quite a jolt.

► **Consider** that when you are trying to heal, your body wants to remain as balanced as possible. For now, put the foods aside that stimulate your body and cause cravings. Once you break the daily cycle of eating these foods, your body will be more likely to gradually stop craving them.

I know how ridiculous this may sound to some; but as a previous chocoholic, I decided to give up the "dark poison" while I was healing and improving my digestive enzymes. I would not believe unless it happened to me; now I rarely if ever crave chocolate. It was amazing. Once I removed the fake, chemically treated foods from my diet, I was able to listen to what my body was really craving—great tasting and nutritious *real* foods.

Replace these dopamine-producing foods with whole foods that digest slower in your system like sprouted grains, maple syrup, and yogurt cheese. Eat something as soon as you get up in the morning and every two hours until you go to bed to stave off cravings for the wrong foods.

Although I never think of carob a substitute for chocolate, this recipe sure satisfies my sweet tooth—without having to turn on the oven.

Carob Fudge Nut Balls	*(serves 12)*
	1 cup hazelnut butter
	1 cup maple syrup
	1 cup carob powder
	1 teaspoon vanilla extract
	¾ cup dried unsweetened coconut

Mix all ingredients except coconut in a medium bowl. Chill for 15 minutes. Form into teaspoon-sized balls and roll in dried coconut. Serve or refrigerate for later.

DIABETES

The origin, mechanisms and progression of diabetes are well understood by the medical community. Aside from individuals who are genetically predisposed, there are millions of people diagnosed with diabetes due to poor diet and lifestyle.

More and more children are being diagnosed with what used to be considered an adult disease, type II diabetes. It is logical to assume that the enormous amount of sugar their bodies attempt to break down every day has overwhelmed their pancreas to the point of malfunction. There is no other logical explanation for this. Yet we continue to eat the same poor quality, sugary, refined foods and expect different results. Ironically, we consume such inordinate amounts of fuel in the form of sugars and yet seem to be lacking the very energy or the initiative to be active and burn our bodies' fuel. Something is very wrong with this picture.

As a society, we keep denying the obvious. Diet and lifestyle have a huge impact on one's health. Diet pills, sugar-free foods and quick fixes have not worked. If we continue to consume chemically infused, processed foods, we will continue to obtain the same results, sickness and disease.

▶ **Consider** that although some people are predisposed and become diabetic, most can avoid this disease with proper diet and exercise.

Quick fixes and prescription medications are not the only options to restore your health. Start by paying attention to what foods you eat. Introduce quinoa, sprouted grains, organic dairy products and more fruits and vegetables into your diet. Eat foods that are full of nutrition and not empty refined calories. If a person is obese or extremely overweight, losing just ten pounds reduces their chance of developing diabetes by up to 60 percent.

An earthshaking thought, perhaps, but you might want to consider that you could take responsibility for your health. Take back your control and allow more sweetness into your emotional, spiritual and intellectual areas of your life as opposed to your diet. Be open to receive the sweetness that life offers to us in many different ways. Sweetness is a wonderful thing.

DIETING

Our "dieting" culture is a huge failure. The concept of dieting became popular fifty years ago and, not so coincidentally, after we began the practices of adding chemicals to our agriculture and processing our food. After fifty years, over two-thirds of our population is either overweight or obese. We are experiencing a serious epidemic of dis-eases spawned from what we eat. An astonishing fact is that the population has gained more weight since reduced-fat products were introduced! We live in a fat-enabling society. We are what we do *not* eat seems to make better sense in this climate of obsessive insanity over our appearance as opposed to our health.

Over 30 billion dollars is spent annually on weight loss and 240 billion dollars is spent on diet-related illnesses: diabetes, cancer, heart problems, indigestion, arthritis, allergies, bowel irregularity, obesity, celiac disease, and autoimmune disorders, to mention just a few.

Diets have not worked; they have just added to the confusion and nutritional schizophrenia that shrouds eating. The Surgeon General stated that obesity is the most pressing public health issue in America. Indeed, it is pressing on the seams of our society in proportion to the medical costs and the stress of psychological damage.

► **Consider** that you can lose your excess weight by eating great tasting, real food that digests easily. This concept is so simple and yet so contrary to the philosophy of our food industry that it boggles the mind. Stop dieting and eat real food that provides nutritious fuel for your body and satisfaction for your palette. Believe me, it is that simple. Never underestimate the power of organic whole food or yourself!

EMOTIONAL NUTRITION

Optimal health is not only about eating healthy foods. Do not forget about your emotional nutrition.

This concept is so simple and yet so contrary to the philosophy of our food industry that it boggles the mind.

► **Consider** taking care of yourself first *and then* your loved ones. Read a good book. Remember, self-love is the only diet aid you will ever really need. Dr. Hong Zhaoguang, author of *Taking the Healthy Train*, believes in "four bests" for creating emotional and mental health: the best doctor is you, the best medicine is time, the best state of mind is peace and the best exercise is walking.

FERTILITY

For the last one hundred years, human fertility has been declining. There is no question about it; the chemicals in our environment have directly affected women's health by disrupting their natural hormonal rhythms and severely compromising their immune systems.

Dioxin, the pollutant responsible for the environmental disasters that occurred at Love Canal, New York, and Times Beach, Missouri, has been found to cause endometriosis in animals. Their endometriosis worsened in relation to the amount of dioxins found in their diet. Endometriosis, a mysterious and painful gynecological and immunological condition, often results in infertility.

Researchers have linked endometriosis to a higher incidence of breast and ovarian cancer, malignant melanoma and auto-immune disorders. Studies have shown that chemicals polluting lakes and swamps in Florida are responsible for birth defects and lower fertility in alligators. Some theorize that pesticides can artificially raise estrogen levels, causing defective eggs in female alligators and smaller genitalia in male alligators.

▶ **Consider** that producing healthy eggs and sperm directly relates to your diet. Eating real foods and getting the chemicals out of your life is of utmost importance if you want to conceive a healthy child. Every step you take will impact your health and the health of your world. Preserve your health and that of your family without preservatives!

Consuming fewer animal products will incredibly decrease your exposure to dioxins. Use organic meat and dairy products as embellishments to your diet, not as staples. When possible, consume local products that do not contain dioxin-contaminated pesticides. Thoroughly wash all vegetables and fruits, even organic produce. Peel waxed produce.

FOOD ALLERGIES

When did food allergies become an accepted daily disease? As more and more chemicals enter our food supply, food allergies will remain a challenge. There are two easy ways to determine if the foods that you are eating are causing you dis-ease, the Mucus Reaction test and the Food Elimination test. For the Mucus Reaction test, simply put the food in question in your mouth and notice the reaction. Does mucus start to excrete in your mouth, do your eyes run, do you sneeze or cough? These are all signals from your body telling you that this food is not for you. Avoiding foods that give you this reaction will allow your body to heal.

▶ **Consider** using the Food Elimination Test for food allergies. Take one food at a time and do not eat it for four days. On the fifth day, eat a small amount of the food in question and notice your reaction. If your body has an allergic reaction or any of the symptoms from the Mucus Reaction test, then you are allergic to this particular food. Often it is the foods you do not think are giving you a problem that fails this test. If you are having difficulty, keep a particular food out of your diet for the four days; it is a sure sign that this is a problem food for you. Start by testing the food ingredients that you may be eating every day like wheat, dairy products and nuts.

If you are allergic to a certain food, it is usually a sign that your body is not healthy enough to digest it. For now, remove the problematic foods from your diet until your body's digestive system is restored to health. The best way to prevent food allergies is to create an essential environment in your body by removing the harmful chemicals from your life and from the food that you eat.

LAUGHING

Laughing lowers your blood sugar which is part of maintaining your overall health. Remember the beloved chimney sweep in Mary Poppins who said, "the more I laugh, the more I'm filled with glee, and the more I laugh, the more I'm a merrier me!" Sounds like logical advice to me!

▶ **Consider** laughing more. I practice laughing when I am alone in my car. Just the act of practicing laughing makes me laugh for real. Then again, I'm unusual, but healthy!

OBESITY

Every day I hear or read something about the obesity epidemic. I know that you too are inundated with the social and physical aspects of the obesity issue. It has surpassed smoking as the top of the list of health issues. So let us look at some solutions for this problem.

▶ **Consider** that a person's diet is the major cause of becoming overweight or obese. We weigh too much, because we eat too much of the wrong foods. Introduce great tasting, easy-to-digest whole foods back into your diet. Foods that are chemical-free and not processed offer the best protection against mindless binge eating and empty calories.

Eat at home. Studies show that we consume up to twice as many calories, fat and sodium when we dine out. Turning off the television and avoid doing other activities while eating at home. This will create mindfulness in eating and slow down your food consumption.

Demonstrate a priceless example for your children the next time you are preparing a meal. Make better food choices and decide on the menu. Children want and need guidance and structured meals. Filling up on healthy foods will help young people naturally avoid junk foods. Help children to understand that making better food choices will empower them to maintain *their* normal weight.

Gather support for your eating lifestyle. Ask friends and family to join you in your quest to get healthy and lose your excess weight. Discuss ways they can help you stay on track.

Get real. Stop the denial that keeps you from taking the next simple step toward ob-

At my peak, I was a size sixteen and have maintained my normal weight of a size six for over ten years. This was accomplished without dieting or deprivation, simply by eating essentially.

taining and maintaining your normal weight. It is possible; I know from experience that it can be a permanent achievement. At my peak, I was a size sixteen and have maintained my normal weight of a size six for over ten years. This was accomplished without dieting or deprivation, simply by eating essentially.

Look at the core foods you eat every week. Start by substituting a whole, real food or recipe for just one of the foods you currently eat that does not support your health. For example, purchase 100 percent sprouted grain bread, as a substitute for regular bread. Sprouted grains digest as a vegetable, not a starch, making them easier for the body to process. (See grains.) Incorporate that food into your eating lifestyle and pick another one. In a few weeks or months, you will be eating more real foods that are preservative and chemical-free. Also, these real foods will be supporting your health and helping you to lose your excess weight. Do not diet or deprive yourself. Instead, eat tasty foods that are real and not processed.

OVER-THE-COUNTER DRUGS

Over-the-counter (OTC) drugs are not without risk. If used improperly they can and do cause serious and sometimes irreparable damage, with the agonizing reality of physical dependence.

▶ **Consider** that manufacturers are capable of and do reformulate their products at higher and lower strengths. Always make sure you read the label and the warnings about side affects and drug combinations. Becoming aware and informed arms us against the casual acceptance of powerful chemicals and narcotics. Selecting an OTC drug should not turn into a game of Russian roulette. Create essential environments by removing harmful chemicals so you do not have to be dependent on drugs.

POSTURE AND EXERCISE

In addition to a healthy diet, your body's posture is important, as well as regular exercise.

▶ **Consider** that your posture affects every part of your body, including digestion. Take a deep breath and stand up straight. The benefits of regular exercise, something as simple as walking, can tremendously improve your health and positively affect how your body absorbs food.

PRESCRIPTION DRUGS

Similar to food manufacturers, drug companies' first goal is to make a profit, not to promote better health. Be aware of health benefits touted by drug companies. Research projects for drugs are often funded by the manufacturers of the very products that are being tested.

The 52 million Americans who need medical intervention for high cholesterol have made Lipitor the best-selling pharmaceutical in history. The cost of organic food should be compared to the cost of prescription drugs. The last time I checked, one of the leading drugs for indigestion cost over $200 for a month's supply. More importantly, organic food does not come with a mile long list of possible interactions.

Without question, a place for prescription drugs does exist, yet our excessive and impatient culture has turned into a population of desperate pink pill poppers. Prescription drugs treat symptoms, not the causes of dis-ease. The two most prescribed drugs today are for indigestion, a symptom preventable by eating foods that taste great and are easy-to-digest. Advertising promotes taking antacids prior to eating certain foods as a precaution to indigestion. Why not avoid indigestion in the first place? If we all accepted the responsibility for our eating habits, who would buy the pink pills?

When on medication, it is even more important to sustain a balanced eating lifestyle.

Over 3 million pounds of antibiotics are prescribed to Americans annually. Antibiotics are often over prescribed when they are not effective. Many are for viral infections such as flu and colds which antibiotics do not address. Over 24 million pounds of antibiotics are fed to animals grown for human consumption. The overuse of antibiotics is making us less and less resistant to antibiotics when they are needed. Investigate other alternative medicines and healing modalities that are available to keep your immune system healthy and reduce your need for antibiotics.

▶ **Consider** that prescription drugs including anti-depressants, anti-inflammatory medications, blood pressure medications, estrogen and tranquilizers may deplete your body of vital minerals and vitamins. When on medication, it is even more important to sustain a balanced eating lifestyle.

Eating a healthy diet rich in organic foods is a lesser expenditure than doctor visits, prescription drugs and daily dis-ease. Drugs cause effects, not side effects. Evaluate the prescription drugs you are taking and consider that by fueling your body better, you could reduce your drug usage. Sorry, there is no such thing as a free lunch or a magical pink pill.

Food Related Topics

FOOD ADVERTISING'S INFLUENCE ON CHILDREN

Babies have a natural instinct at birth to know when their stomachs are full. This natural instinct makes them push away their mother's breast or bottle when they have had enough food. By the time they are of school age, the effects of the outside world causes children to stop listening to this inner instinct. This has been largely due to the omnipresent intrusion of television into their consciousness.

Twelve billion dollars is spent each year to promote and sponsor foods to children. On an average, young children watch over four hours of television per day. The message is clear that a trend to eat more frequently, to eat more convenience foods and to eat larger proportions has become a daily routine of unhealthy proportions. Children succumb to advertising pressure from television that promotes high-fat, high-caloric and chemically-laden foods. And the crime is that our society revolves around the fallacy that it cannot be that bad; unfortunately they are right, *it is worse*.

Kids spend two billion dollars of their money on snack foods annually—more than anything else including clothing, books and entertainment. The average American child views about 10,000 food ads per year, an average of over 27 per day. It is no wonder that 25 percent of our children are currently overweight or obese, with many more headed in that direction. With weight problems, lack of any structured exercise and refined snacks, the early onset of diabetes is inevitable and yet, sadly, most times avoidable.

In Italy, Australia, Norway and Sweden, advertising is prohibited on children's television shows. However, at the present time in the United States, there are no laws prohibiting food ads from being aired during children's programming. In fact, many schools utilize closed circuit television systems that impart more exposure to ads in the faux format of supposed educational benefit. And the real clincher is that most large snack food companies gladly sponsor the purchase of the video equipment for the schools. Sounds like insider advertising to me! Banning all ads for children under the age of eight was proposed in the 1970s. Both powerful and controlling, the food, advertising and broadcasting industries stopped the much needed ban from becoming law.

▶ **Consider** that limiting your child's television exposure could save them from a great deal of the pressures experienced from food advertising. Start at an early age by educating your child about healthy foods. Believe it or not, children are not naturally drawn to a lot of sugar. They develop this craving and become accustomed to having it in their diet. Consider limiting the sugars and additives your children are exposed to by incorporating a little cooking into your family activities. Invite your children to help in the purchase and preparation of the healthy food choices. Natural fruits and veggies are good but remember children also need good fats, healthy protein and exercise to develop strong bodies.

Education is the key. Buy a fast-food cheeseburger or a donut and let it sit on your kitchen counter. Mine has been in a plastic container traveling around the country with me for the last three years and it has not changed. No rot, no mold, and no decay. It is a great visual for children to see what happens or does not happen to food that is processed. Sprouting some seeds in a jar on your counter will help children understand how real food is grown. Plant a garden. Discuss how nearly all food manufacturers use the power of advertising to entice children to spend money, not to get healthy. Show your children organic produce in the grocery store and how natural it looks compared to conventionally grown produce. Real food has blemishes and that is a good thing! Children are often smarter, more perceptive and open to change than we give them credit for. Try it. They are worth it!

Show your children organic produce in the grocery store and how natural it looks compared to conventionally grown produce. Real food has blemishes and that is a good thing!

THREE SQUARES

The traditional concept of eating three square meals a day, breakfast, lunch and dinner, might not restore or maintain your health quite as much as eating every two hours. If more than two hours are allowed to pass in between meals, your body's blood sugar and metabolism can become unbalanced.

▶ **Consider** eating smaller meals or snacks throughout the day in order to keep your metabolism balanced and your hunger at bay. Eating snacks such as a half sandwich, a few dried apricots, some yogurt, or a banana in between meals can improve your digestion more than the good old three squares.

YOUR FIRE

You are smarter than you think. We all virtually know what constitutes real food and what does not. You know that sewer sludge fertilizer, fake juices, irradiated meats, and flavor-filled, chemically-processed foods are not the path to better health. Do not allow the nutritional confusion and in-your-face convenience foods prevent you from seizing responsibility for your health. You can start right now by making better food choices to restore and maintain your health. You are worth it. Life is worth it.

There are many good people out there widening the path to a better food supply: Todd Murphy, creator and owner of the Farmer's Diner in Vermont; Susan and Alan Bullock of Back Achers Farm, are setting the standard for sustainable farmers everywhere; Jeff Smeltzer, an organic farmer in Northeastern Pennsylvania who is dedicated to growing organic spelt and Dr. Peter and Janie Brodhead, owners of Brighter Day Natural Foods in Savannah, Georgia have been making it easier for people to better their lives and environments. Support these and other entrepreneurs and the socially responsible businesses they represent.

Specific Foods

BEVERAGES

Alcoholic beverages. Alcohol is a food and just like other foods, it can be and is abused, thereby resulting in impaired judgment that translates into massive health costs. In addition to its many drawbacks, most alcoholic beverages contain added or naturally occurring substances that some bodies cannot easily digest such as tannins, histamines and sulfites. Just like other foods, chemicals are used in growing the crops that are distilled into alcohols. A quick glance at the beverage's label provides a WARNING: Drinking distilled spirits: beer, wine, coolers and other alcoholic beverages may increase cancer risk and during pregnancy can cause birth defects. It certainly sounds straightforward to me.

▶ **Consider** recognizing the effects of alcohol, or other food and drugs that destroy the quality of your health. If you are experiencing allergic reactions such as a flushed face or headaches, avoid alcohol until your digestive system heals and can more easily digest these substances.

Breast milk & baby formula. Although there is no substitute for human milk, it is the most chemically contaminated human food available today. Dioxins, cleaning fluids, insect poisons, dry cleaning fluids, lead, flame retardants, Polychlorinated Biphenyls (PCBs), mercury and other chemicals are common contaminants found in a mother's breast milk. Not so yummy. An average breastfed infant ingests fifty times more PCBs per pound of body weight than an adult.

On the other hand, baby formula can contain contaminants from the manufacturing process. They may also contain excessive levels of metals, including cadmium, lead, aluminum and manganese. Soy formulas result in a high level of plant-derived estrogens (photoestrogens) found in infants. Understand that baby formula is an $8-billion-dollar-a-year industry that commits huge advertising budgets to sway more and more women off the idea of breastfeeding. What industry is promoting breastfeeding? None.

▶ **Consider** that despite the problems with persistent chemicals, nursing for most women is still a better choice than formula. The levels of chemicals in most women are not high enough to outweigh the hazards of infant formula. Protecting a baby against diabetes, obesity and certain cancers and juvenile arthritis are a few of the benefits of breastfeeding. Breast milk is alive and a better choice than baby formula for the development of your child.

The levels of chemicals in most women are not high enough to outweigh the hazards of infant formula.

In cases when a mother is unable to produce enough breast milk or, for medical reasons, cannot breastfeed her infant, baby formula can be improved by adding some real food and vitamin ingredients. First choose a baby formula with the least amount of chemicals. Enhance the digestibility by using 1 part yogurt and 3 parts water to dilute the formula. Liquid vitamins and minerals can also be added. Mother and child health experts, Mary Bove, N.D. and Aviva Romm offer these and many other commonsense, natural solutions. (See Sources.)

Bear in mind the importance of creating an essential environment and of removing the chemicals from your body and home before you plan to conceive a child. This will benefit you, your baby and your family.

During pregnancy, some of the other risks to avoid are alcoholic beverages and tobacco products (and its smoke). Avoid using pesticides, solvents, paints, non-water-based glues, and harsh, non-biodegradable cleaning products. Avoid dry cleaned clothes. Avoid exposure to gasoline fumes, nail polish and polish remover. Avoid eating animal fats and high-fat dairy products. Eat organic food and avoid fish that may contain higher levels of PCBs and mercury.

The choice to breastfeed has an added benefit for the environment in that it reduces the use of our resources and chemicals used in the production of baby formula. For more information on this issue visit the Natural Resources Defense Council website at www.nrdc.org/breastmilk.

Coffee. Following oil, coffee is the second largest import in the United States. Americans consume an average of 400,000,000 cups of coffee per day. Due to the high demand for coffee, farmers are being put out of business and are being replaced by "green deserts" managed by agribusiness. These are farms where native forests have been cleared and replaced with rows of short coffee trees that get drenched with chemical cocktails of fertilizers, pesticides and herbicides. The results are tragic. Prices have plummeted to all-time lows and many small farmers are not able to maintain their land or to provide for their families because they are being driven into a cycle of poverty and debt. Agricultural workers are being exposed to toxic chemicals, native and migratory bird habitats are being destroyed, the water supply is being contaminated and pesticide poisoning is being imported from other parts of the world—and coffee drinkers are the recipients.

▶ **Consider** that Fair Trade was developed as the solution to this crisis. Fair Trade assures consumers that the coffee we drink was purchased under fair conditions. Certified Fair Trade importers must meet strict international guidelines, paying a minimum price per pound. This provides the much needed resources to the farmers who could use assistance in transitioning to and maintaining less toxic growing methods.

Buy coffee with the Certified Fair Trade logo. The result will make you feel good for many reasons—better community development, health, education, and environmental stewardship. Now that you know there is a conscious choice, you can make a better one.

Milk. Milk has been reported to be the number one food responsible for more allergies than any other food. The dairy industry is subsidized by the Federal Government which accounts for the artificially low price of milk. Faced with an obesity epidemic of unparalleled proportions, our tax dollars would be better spent, other than a multi-million dollar advertising campaign to push milk. If milk is so good for us, why does the dairy industry and the government elect to spend millions on print, radio, television and outdoor advertising, often using highly paid celebrities, to sell this product to us? Why not use these advertising dollars to promote vegetables such as, spinach or green beans? Do not get me started! And, for goodness sakes, wipe that milk mustache off your face! Got Spinach?

▶ **Consider** that there are other ways to get calcium rich foods into your diet. It is not the lack of milk in your diet, but the lack of a *healthy* diet that could lead to osteoporosis. Some of the nutritious foods that contain calcium are almonds, asparagus, blackstrap molasses, broccoli, cabbage, carob, kale, kelp, oats, prunes, sesame seeds, soybeans, figs, and filberts. Herbs such as alfalfa, burdock root, cayenne, flaxseed, horsetail, kelp, nettle, paprika, parsley, peppermint, raspberry leaves, red clover, rose hips and yarrow also contain calcium. Calcium supplements are an option, but please, read the label first or consult with your doctor. For those skeptics who remain unconvinced, ponder the estimated 82 different drugs used in conventional dairy farming.

Soft Drinks. Lawmakers in several states are pushing legislation to help Americans consume healthier drinks. A movement is underway to discontinue the sale of soft drinks in schools. Legislation targeted at ridding schools of soft drinks and foods that are high in sugar content is being faced with strong opposition from the National Soft Drink Association. One of the major soda companies fills 4.5 billion cans of soda a day with ingredients such as chemicals, additives and sugar. Then imagine the number of young people who fill themselves up every day with these easily accessible and unhealthy products. Visualize the triumph of getting these unwholesome temptations out of our schools.

The good news is that California has banned soft drinks in schools and many states are considering following suit. When soft drinks are removed from our schools, it sends a powerful message to our children about the effects of unhealthy foods. Children crave guidance and they learn by example.

Soft drinks do not provide healthy fuel for your body and their harmful chemicals get trapped and stored in your cells. Sounds lovely, does it not? If you are trying to lose weight or restore your health, soft drinks surely will not help you achieve that goal. Diet soft drinks, promoted as an oasis for the calorie challenged individual, can be a nasty brew of vile chemicals that appallingly are not listed on the container. Ironically, diet sodas, meant for those who are trying to rid their body of excess weight and toxicity, can actually add more of the same. Human bodies are not programmed to digest diet or any other kind of soft drink, which are nothing more than sugar-laden, chemical-flavored, colored water. I guess they call them soft drinks since they have a tendency to make us soft in the middle.

Soft drinks do not fit the criteria for real food— food that is chemical free, organic in nature, in-season and easy-to-digest.

▶ **Consider** when choosing beverages, that soft drinks do not fit the criteria for real food—food that is chemical free, organic in nature, in-season and easy-to-digest. Instead, try refreshing herbal tea or vegetable juice. Spring water is always a good substitute for colored, sugar-filled drinks. Squeeze a little juice from a fresh lemon or orange into your spring water and voila, you are safe sipping in style.

Try this recipe for a refreshingly, safe and nutritious drink.

Cranberry Juice	(serves 8)
	4 cups 100% cranberry juice
	4 cups water
	¾ cup maple syrup

Pour a 32-ounce jar of cranberry juice into a large pitcher. Fill the empty jar with water and pour into the pitcher. Add maple syrup and stir. Chill and serve. If desired, dilute with additional water to taste. The syrup can also be adjusted to your taste. Cranberries digest as vegetables, so this drink is easy for your body to process.

CHEWING GUM

Chewing gum can have a very soothing and calming effect; actually that fact is one of the habit's positive aspects. On the negative side, anything you put into your mouth and chew sends a message to the brain to release digestive enzymes into the stomach. As a result of this false alarm, chewing gum has the potential to cause stomach upset or hunger pangs.

Aspartame, a common ingredient found in chewing gum and in diet sodas is dangerous to your health. The prominent side affects associated with aspartame consumption are headaches, dizziness, confusion, memory loss, panic attacks, chest pains, birth defects, erratic heart beats, burning urine and others.

▶ **Consider** reading the ingredients on gum labels. Although aspartame is still considered a safe food additive by some, why take the risk? Chew gum that does not contain aspartame. There are several aspartame-free and satisfying chewing gums that are on the market, available mostly at health food stores. Although chewing gum can be enjoyable, it would be wise to limit this activity to assure your digestive system does not work overtime. Do not get stuck on it!

CORN

Since 1930 the United States has increased corn production from around 2 billion bushels to almost 10 billion bushels annually. Corn is the most subsidized farm product at approximately 5 billion per year. The use of corn syrup and corn oil has increased 4,000 percent in the last 50 years. Corn is in thousands of the products we consume daily. Some say we are being "cornified."

Low-priced corn has been the building block of the fast-food industry. Corn by-products like high-fructose corn syrup have made possible the super sizing of soda. Cheap corn fed to cattle has allowed fast food to provide cheap, oversized hamburgers. Cheap corn has fueled the explosion of highly processed foods at a rate of 10,000 new products a year. Even chicken nuggets are corn-based, from the corn-fed chicken to the corn binding and bulking agents that hold them together. When food is inexpensive and abundant, people will naturally eat more with the inevitable and unnatural consequences of becoming both fat and unhealthy. Americans consume three times more corn sweetener than any other kind of sweetener. It is practically in everything, either directly or indirectly.

Free-range chickens that are fed organic feed lay happy eggs.

The easiest and most lucrative thing to do with cheap, abundant crops is to turn them into foods like corn sweetener, corn feed, and highly processed foods that are more profitable than the crop in its original form. Keep in mind that agriculture is not about the food, or the farming, or the consumers; it is about the money. From the amber waves of grain, the 1960's Green Revolution created a new crop called cash!

▶ **Consider** that you are smarter than this. Become aware of the "value-added," processed foods that are contributing to this broad state of dis-ease. Avoid super-sized portions. Steer clear of foods that are laced with trans-fats and sugar. Buy baked organic corn chips, organic frozen corn, organic corn pasta and foods that are not processed. The avalanche of cheap grain derived products need not devastate your good health.

EGGS

For many years, eggs had a bad reputation, but recently have been redeemed as a great whole food. However, unless they are organic, they can be nasty. I purchased several dozen regular supermarket eggs to see what kind of shelf life they might have. They last a few months without going bad versus organic eggs that last a couple of weeks. When anything lasts that long, it takes your appetite away.

▶ **Consider** buying eggs that are laid by happy chickens. Free-range chickens that are fed organic feed lay happy eggs. They are not caged up and fed chemicals, growth hormones or antibiotics. In addition, who decided that packaging eggs in plastic containers was a good idea? It is just another place of being innocently exposed to further toxicity in our daily routines or habits. Buy organic eggs, preferably in paper cartons. There is nothing like a fresh egg.

FISH & SHELLFISH

Groundwater contamination which is caused by pesticide run-off has spread pollutants to our rivers, lakes and oceans. In the Gulf of Mexico, the chemical residue of pesticides and fertilizers from the Mississippi River has caused a dead spot the size of New Jersey. These pollutants are absorbed and consumed by fish, wildlife and aquatic plants. Just like other foods, we need to know where our fish is grown and what it was fed.

Farm-raised fish, mostly salmon, has become popular due to its profitability, not because of its health benefits. Although mercury levels were roughly the same, studies illustrate that most farm-raised fish contain more harmful chemicals, more Polychlorinated Biphenyls (PCBs), more dioxins, more fat, and significantly less beneficial omega-3 fatty acids. Most of the methods used in farm-raised salmon include the use of chemical additives, pesticides, colorings and fungicides that contribute to the pollution of our resources.

Eating fish from unknown sources can increase your exposure to pollutants, like dioxin, that come from soil runoff and industrial air pollution. These dioxins and other harmful chemicals collect in the fatty tissue of both fish and animals. When fish is eaten from polluted waters, it increases your risk of these chemicals entering your body. Fish that contains higher levels of mercury from polluted waters include shark, swordfish, King mackerel, canned albacore tuna and tilefish.

Shellfish, such as lobster and shrimp are high in cholesterol and are one of the hardest foods for the human body to break down and to process. It takes an enormous amount of digestive enzymes to digest shellfish. To restore your digestive health, eat fish that does not live in a shell.

▶ **Consider** that you do not have to stop eating fish. Until safer standards are implemented, choose other alternatives. Consume other fish that are not endangered or depleted which are good sources of omega-3 fats including haddock, flounder, sole, striped bass, mahi-mahi, whitefish, Pacific cod and Pacific halibut. Eat a variety of fish and limit your intake of farm-raised salmon to once or twice a month, unless you know the farm or the supplier and can verify their growing practices.

Get to know your fish supplier and request organic or wild fish selections. Ask grocers and waiters questions to find out where the fish was caught. Do not be shy. Go ahead and smell the fish you buy; fresh fish *does not* smell fishy. Avoid buying fish that is wrapped in plastic; do not buy what you are not able to smell or perhaps what they do not want you to smell. Buy fish that has been nature-raised when possible. The good news is that new labeling will be required for fish indicating where it was caught, processed and whether it is wild or farmed.

When preparing fish, broil or bake on a rack thereby causing any pollutants stored in the fat to drip away. Avoid deep-fried fish as it seals in the pollutants. Read the label on canned fish such as tuna and salmon, and purchase those that do not contain salt and are packed in spring water, not oil. In addition, buy tuna fish that is all natural with the dolphin-safe logo.

Try this recipe for an easy, nutritious entree.

Herb Baked Fish	(serves 4)
	1½ pounds flounder (4–6 filets)
	¼ cup melted butter
	¼ cup fresh lemon juice
	½ cup vegetable broth or water
	1 teaspoon dill weed
	½ teaspoon onion powder
	1 teaspoon dried oregano
	½ teaspoon paprika
	Salt and pepper to taste

Preheat oven to 450 degrees. Place fish in a greased, shallow baking dish. Melt butter in a small saucepan over low heat. Stir in remaining ingredients and spread mixture evenly over the fish. Sprinkle extra paprika over the top of fish. Bake uncovered 10–15 minutes, until fish is done.

FRUITS & VEGETABLES

Produce travels an average distance of 1500 miles before it arrives at the grocery store. To travel great distances, produce is often picked four to seven days before it reaches the store shelf. Be aware that fruits and vegetables begin to lose flavor and nutrients as soon as they are picked.

Because they are picked prior to ripening, conventionally grown fruits and vegetables are sometimes gassed to induce ripening. You have probably purchased fruit such as peaches or apples that looked absolutely perfect on the outside, but upon biting into them, discover that they are pretty tasteless. And since they never really spoil, they continue to disappoint us with regard to taste and nutritional value. This is compounded by the threat of deadly chemicals which have been added to the growing process.

We are rearing an entire generation to expect and accept the fact that fruits and vegetables go from green to rotten with very little taste in between. What has happened to the delicious riped fruit? The produce market has developed into a premature holding cell for fruits and vegetables that never became what they were intended to be—pure, tasty and nourishing.

▶ **Consider** buying organic fruits and vegetables that are in-season and locally grown whenever available to reduce the use of our natural resources and to protect your health. Buying a larger variety of fruits and vegetables will encourage growers to diversify their crops. Try a new fruit or vegetable each month or each week, such as pumpkin, red peppers, wild rice, sweet potatoes, eggplant, avocados or strawberries. Vegetables retain more nutrients when they are steamed versus boiled.

Do not forget that even organic fruits and vegetables need to be washed. Fruit and vegetable wash is sold in stores, but I prefer to use a solution of a little baking soda and water. In a clean sink add 2–3 tablespoons of baking soda. Immerse vegetables or fruit and wash. Do not wash fruits and vegetables before storing them.

You can also make your own bottled produce wash solution. It is less expensive and does not add another plastic bottle to your grocery list and the landfill. If you already have a plastic bottle, create your own veggie wash by filling it with water and adding a few drops of liquid chemical-free dish soap.

The University of Tennessee conducted a study of 56 girls between the ages of 8 to 13 and found that those who ate at least 3 servings of fruits and vegetables a day had bigger bones than their peers. This shows that fruits and vegetables, not just dairy, are important in strengthening bones.

Introduce more vegetables into your eating lifestyle with this easy to make, tasty soup.

Wheat-free Tortilla Soup	*(serves 6)*
	1 tablespoon butter
	1/3 cup chopped onions
	2 cloves garlic, chopped
	1 small diced green or red chili (hot or mild), chopped
	5 large fresh tomatoes, chopped (or a 14-ounce can of diced)
	1 teaspoon dried oregano
	3/4 teaspoon ground cumin
	1/8 teaspoon chili powder
	1/4 teaspoon pepper
	8 cups vegetable or chicken broth
	10 corn tortillas
	1 ripe avocado
	2 tablespoons chopped fresh cilantro or parsley
	1 cup corn kernels
	Sour cream to garnish

Heat a 6-quart pan over medium heat. Melt butter and add onion, garlic, chili, oregano, cumin, chili powder and pepper; sauté 1 minute. Add broth and tomatoes (including juice). Cover and bring to a simmer over medium-high heat. Stack tortillas and cut into 1/8-inch strips. Add tortillas to simmering broth. Reduce heat, cover and simmer 15 minutes, stirring occasionally. Peel, pit, and coarsely chop the avocado. Add avocado to soup with corn, cilantro or parsley and heat. Serve garnished with a teaspoon of sour cream—organic, of course.

GRAINS: CARBOHYDRATES, SPROUTED GRAINS TO THE RESCUE & WHEAT PRODUCTS

Carbohydrates. Our culture is producing a lot of "carbophobes." Even people who do not understand the function of carbohydrates are avoiding them!

Scientifically, all carbohydrates fall into the same category. Carbohydrates include some fruits, some vegetables and starches. They are foods that the body quickly turns into digestible sugars. Because you want to keep your body balanced through proper digestion, it is important to differentiate between starches and carbohydrates as there is a big difference in their digestibility.

Fruit and vegetable carbohydrates are broken down and digested by the body using vegetable enzymes. Starches, such as wheat, rice and other grains, require pancreatic enzymes to breakdown and digest properly. The reason it is easier for most people to digest fruit and vegetable carbohydrates versus starch carbohydrates is that the body produces an abundant amount of vegetable enzymes, but not a large amount of pancreatic enzymes.

▶ **Consider** eating carbohydrates that digest like fruits and vegetables, not starches. Complex carbohydrates such as fruits, vegetables and *sprouted* grains are better for you and easier to digest than simple carbohydrates such as wheat and other grains. *Sprouted* grains are complex carbohydrates that use vegetable enzymes to break down and they digest slowly in the body. Remember, some fruits and vegetables, such as corn and potatoes are considered carbohydrates or starchy vegetables, but they *still* digest like vegetables, not starches.

Sprouted grains to the rescue. Sprouted grain products were the key to restoring my health, losing my excess weight and creating a stress-free environment in my body. Being able to eat breads, crackers, cakes, muffins, cookies and waffles made with 100 percent sprouted grain flour enabled me to follow a healthy eating lifestyle. When a grain is sprouted, it changes the composition of the starch molecules, converting them into vegetable sugars, so the body recognizes and digests sprouted grains as a vegetable. Picture a wheat seed; as it grows into grass it changes from a starch into a vegetable. Sprouting grains that are then milled into flour is the same concept. With so many options, it is foolish to tax your digestive system needlessly.

▶ **Consider** that you can start today by replacing your wheat bread and wheat products with sprouted bread, sprouted flours and sprouted grain products. One hundred percent sprouted bread is sold at health food stores and some grocery stores. The Essential Eating Sprouted Flour Company, the first certified organic sprouted mill in the country, offers sprouted spelt flour, sprouted wheat flour, sprouted rye flour and sprouted cream of spelt cereal. (See Sources.) Sprouted grains can be traced back to pre-biblical times. Our vision is to bring sprouted products back into our culture, a vision of which we can all be a part.

Eat sprouted grain bread and use sprouted flour in your baking. It can be substituted one for one in your recipes that use bread and white flour. This will allow your body to heal and to increase your production of pancreatic enzymes. Over time you can reintroduce unsprouted grains back into your diet, but even then, bodies never want large amounts and always prefer sprouted grains.

Still in need of further persuading? All right then, nibble on this tasty fact: sprouted grains create enzymes that *actually aid* in digestion. Breaking down the complex sugars can help eliminate painful gas, and increase vitamin and mineral absorption levels. Sprouting neutralizes the powerful carcinogens and enzyme inhibitors, as well as acid known to inhibit the absorption of calcium, magnesium, iron, copper and zinc.

Try this recipe made with sprouted spelt flour.

Banana Bread

6 tablespoons melted butter
½ cup maple syrup
2 large eggs
4 ripe mashed bananas
1 cup sprouted spelt flour
1 cup cornmeal
1 teaspoon baking soda
1 teaspoon baking powder
½ teaspoon salt

Preheat oven to 375 degrees. In a large mixing bowl, blend butter and syrup. Add eggs and bananas. Mix in remaining ingredients. Pour into greased loaf pan. Bake for 35–45 minutes until it tests done. If using muffin tins, bake 16–18 minutes.

Wheat products. The Standard American Diet (S.A.D.) is wheat-based. Wheat is another one of the hardest-to-digest foods. Not that wheat is a bad food, we just eat entirely too much of it. Cookies, crackers, breads, muffins, cakes, tortillas, pasta, cereal, and many other foods that we consume daily contain wheat.

When a body cannot digest wheat or the digestive tract cannot absorb food digestive disorders occur. Crohn's, colitis, and celiac disease are becoming more and more common among Americans. These diseases are shedding light on the fact that in addition to removing the chemicals from our foods, we need to expand the variety of foods that we eat. Try supplementing your diet with a healthy substitution for each of the harmful subtractions.

▶ **Consider** introducing other nutritious, "grain-type" foods into your diet such as quinoa, polenta pasta, wild rice, sprouted grain flour and sprouted breads. Polenta is ground corn which is a vegetable and wild rice is a grass which is also a vegetable. As mentioned previously, sprouting a grain converts the starch molecules into vegetable sugars. Vegetable sugars digest slowly and do not require pancreatic enzymes.

Sprouted flour and sprouted grains contain only a slight amount of gluten. Gluten is the vegetable protein of a grain, which most people can digest with ease. Many people, unable to digest gluten, are diagnosed as being gluten intolerant when in reality they are actually wheat or starch intolerant. One hundred percent sprouted bread can be purchased at health food stores and some grocery stores.

Sprouted spelt flour can be substituted for recipes using white flour. Try this delicious waffle recipe.

Wheat-free Waffles

2 large eggs
1/4 cup plain yogurt
1 1/4 cups water
3 tablespoons melted butter
1/4 cup maple syrup
1 tablespoon vanilla extract
2 cups sprouted spelt flour
1/2 teaspoon salt
1 tablespoon baking powder

In a large mixing bowl, lightly beat eggs. Add yogurt, water, melted butter, syrup, and vanilla. Mix until smooth. Add the remaining dry ingredients to the egg mixture and mix well. Follow waffle iron instructions for cooking. Adjust consistency of batter by adding more water or flour as needed. Serve with butter and maple syrup.

HYDROGENATED OILS & TRANS FATS

During the hydrogenation process of oils, hydrogen is bubbled through hot vegetable oil in the presence of metal at high temperatures. This significantly alters the oil and gives it a longer shelf life than healthy oils such as olive oil or grape seed oil. Hydrogenation creates trans fat or trans fatty acids that raise the "bad cholesterol" and lowers the "good cholesterol" in the body.

Trans fats are found in foods such as margarine, shortening, most peanut butter and microwaved popcorn. The majority of processed foods such as cookies, frozen breakfast foods, chips and cake mixes are likely to contain trans fat. Since modern food processing bestowed upon us hydrogenated oils, we have witnessed the decline in the usage of healthy fats. Not surprisingly, heart and other related diseases including diabetes have increased.

Trans fat is by far the deadliest fat in the American diet, even worse than saturated fat. Due to recent laws requiring trans fats to be listed on food labels by 2006, the food industry is racing to find a fat free-oil. It will probably result in more biotechnology, more processing and more chemicals. Do not buy into this.

Just like eggs, meat tastes better when it comes from animals that have had a humane life.

▶ **Consider** using healthy oils that are not refined, chemically processed or unnatural. Organic, cold-pressed, extra-virgin olive oil and grape seed oil are the two most nutritious and easiest oils to digest. Organic butter is the very easiest fat to digest. Essential fatty acids are "good" fats and necessary for daily cell function. They lower cholesterol and play a part in the treatment of arthritis. Essential fatty acids can also be obtained from eating such foods as leafy green vegetables, wild salmon, flaxseeds, nuts, sprouted beans and legumes.

The important thing to remember is that healthy fats will not get stuck in your arteries and will be eliminated more easily by the body. The more familiar canola, safflower, soy and corn oils are harder for the body to process, and are widely used because they are less expensive.

When dining out, ask restaurant waiters and cooks what oils are being used. If consuming fewer calories is desired, broth or water can be substituted for oil when sautéing foods. As stated before, we consume 50 percent more fat when dining out. To reduce hydrogenated and hidden oils when dining out, stay away from foods described with the words creamed, crispy, breaded, fritters, batter-dipped, tempura, Alfredo, béarnaise, au gratin and hollandaise.

MEAT & POULTRY

Due to human health risks, the European Union has announced a permanent ban on beef cattle which have been given synthetic growth hormones. In the United States 94 percent of beef cattle have growth hormones implanted in their ears. This debate will go on and on, but concern will be alleviated when the public is made aware that organic beef prohibits the use of hormones or other synthetic chemicals which may cause you dis-ease. Why risk dis-ease from the meat you consume?

Feeding human snack food to livestock has become a common practice. Surpluses of potato chips, pretzels, party mix and popcorn are actually fed to livestock. If it were not so sad, it might be humorous. These snacks fatten up humans, and logically they will do the same to cattle. The chemicals from these foods are stored in the fat of the animal and passed along to you, the consumer, a bonus that we can all do without.

This true story illustrates how chemicals have become an integral part of our meat and poultry production. A friend of mine was hired to paint the chicken coops on a farm. He noticed that there were flies all over and inside his truck, but not in the chicken barns. The farmer explained to him that the chickens are fed insecticides and their insecticide-infested manure keeps the flies away. Scary but true! Now, if only the insecticide-infested meat would keep us away.

▶ **Consider** buying organic meat and poultry that is labeled antibiotic, hormone and chemical-free. Get to know your local butcher. Find out where your meats are grown, how they are raised and what they are fed. Just like eggs, meat tastes better when it comes from animals that have had a humane life.

To avoid bacteria from meat, thoroughly wash surfaces that come in contact with raw meats specifically hands, utensils, cutting boards, sinks and countertops.

POPCORN

You would think that popcorn would be a relatively safe, whole food. I did until I read a report linking a severe lung disease to factory workers handling artificial butter flavoring.

▶ **Consider** that artificial butter flavoring is made from chemicals that are, for the most part, untested and are not required to be disclosed on packaging. Movie popcorn or prepackaged popcorn containing chemicals is not beneficial to your health. Buy organic popcorn and pop it yourself. Pour a little melted organic butter on the top and voila. It is easy and it assures your safety from toxic chemicals.

POTATOES

Monitor and other insecticides used to develop perfect and unblemished crops for fast-food manufacturing and grocery stores, are so noxious that after spraying potatoes, a farmer will stay out of that field for 4–5 days to avoid toxic exposure. Monitor has been found to cause neurological damage to humans. In Idaho, where almost a third of the nation's potatoes are grown, the chemicals added to agriculture are commonly found in groundwater wells and streams. Chemicals and biotechnology allow potatoes to be grown to French-fry perfection, not nutritional perfection.

Most farmers feel bad about using chemicals on their crops, but are compelled to do so because of economics and intense pest pressure. Farmers use chemicals as a labor-saving device that eases the tight profit margins associated with growing food. Regrettably, the application of chemicals to American fields has made them virtually sterile and unsustainable. While the farmer forces himself to use chemicals in order to support his family, he is, in the long run, hurting his family, himself, and every person who sits down to the table to eat. An agribusiness potato farmer confessed to a *New York Times* journalist that he plants a small area of potatoes without chemicals for his personal consumption.

Organic potato farmers use good timing, crop rotation and a little resourcefulness to avoid adding toxic chemicals to our food. Support them.

▶ **Consider** buying organic potatoes. Perhaps you are fortunate enough to be able to grow your own or to be acquainted with a farmer that grows chemical-free potatoes. Organic potato farmers use good timing, crop rotation and a little resourcefulness to avoid adding toxic chemicals to our food. Support them.

Just as it is possible to taste the difference, you can also definitely see the difference between chemically-grown and organic produce. Potatoes that have been grown without toxic pesticides and fertilizers will have imperfections and vary in size—that's a good thing. Offered the choice, I would rather have brown spots and irregularities on my produce than on my body!

Try this recipe using organic potatoes.

Vegetable Mashed Potatoes	(serves 4)
	1 tablespoon butter
	2 leeks, white and light green part only, cut into 1-inch slices
	2 large russet potatoes (1 pound), peeled and cubed
	1 parsnip, peeled and cut into 1-inch pieces
	1 cup spinach, chopped or torn into small pieces
	1 teaspoon oregano
	1 teaspoon salt
	1/4 teaspoon pepper

In a medium saucepan, melt the butter and add leeks, potatoes, parsnips, carrots, oregano, salt and pepper. Add enough water to barely cover vegetables. Bring to a boil, partially covered, over high heat. Reduce the heat and simmer covered, for 10 minutes. Uncover and simmer for 10–15 minutes longer, until the vegetables are fork tender. During the last 5 minutes of cooking the vegetables, add the spinach without stirring, cover and cook until wilted. Drain water off of the vegetables saving 1 cup of the liquid. Using a potato masher, mash vegetables to desired consistency, using reserved liquid to thin as needed. Serve hot.

QUINOA

Quinoa (keen-wa), the mother grain of the Inca Indians, has been around for thousands of years. It fell out of favor primarily because it was not as economical to grow and to harvest as wheat. The beauty of quinoa is two fold; it is an herb that performs like a grain and it is also a complete protein that digests like a fruit. Now, how is that for a great food?

In addition to containing important minerals such as calcium and iron, quinoa is a good source of protein. It looks like couscous when cooked and is very delicious. Organic quinoa is sold in grain, flour and flake form—it is wheat- and gluten-free.

▶ **Consider** eating more quinoa and quinoa pasta, great replacements for wheat and starches. Also, try Vegetable Quinoa Pilaf. Imagine the possibilities!

Vegetable Quinoa Pilaf	(serves 6)
	2 cups quinoa
	1 tablespoon butter
	1 cup grated carrots
	1 bunch fresh spinach
	(or 10 ounce box frozen), chopped
	1 cup chopped chives or onions
	½ cup yogurt cheese or sour cream

Place 4 cups of water or broth in a sauce pan. Add 2 cups of quinoa and bring to a boil. Simmer for 15–17 minutes until quinoa is tender—a little white ring will be visible on the edge of the quinoa grain, let cool. In a large sauté pan, melt butter over medium heat. Add carrots (and onions) and sauté until tender about 6 minutes. Add spinach; cover and steam 5–7 minutes. If vegetables begin to stick, add broth or water a tablespoon at a time. Add cooked quinoa, chives and cheese to vegetable mixture; mix well. Serve warm, chilled or at room temperature.

SOY PRODUCTS

It is called soy milk because bean milk really does not sound all that tasty and you probably would not buy it. Soy products, including soy milk, are derived from soy beans. Soy milk sounds so much more appealing than bean milk, but it is *still* bean milk. Beans are virtually impossible for the human body to break down. It takes an incredibly healthy digestive system not to experience any ill effects from unsprouted beans and soy products. So why are so many soy products being marketed today? Because soy beans are cheap to grow and they have a long shelf life. Soy bean oil is the largest source of added fat to our diet and is also the oil most often found in processed foods.

▶ **Consider** substituting yogurt milk, almond, or cashew milk for soy milk. Stay away from unsprouted soy based products that promise health benefits. A large increase in the public's soy consumption was the result of being informed that Asian women develop less breast cancer because they eat soy. And yet, even though we now consume more soy, our cancers are still not going away.

If you desire the benefits of the dis-ease fighting photo chemicals inherent in soy products, choose fresh soybeans in the pod. Called edamame, they are a great source of protein while doubling as a great snack or salad garnish. They can be found in the frozen section of grocery stores. Many Japanese restaurants serve them as an appetizer. Dried soy beans can also be sprouted, converting them back into vegetables that are easy to digest.

There are more nutritious and healthier alternatives in order to incorporate sufficient quantities of protein and essential amino acids into your eating lifestyle such as quinoa, yogurt, sprouted beans, nuts, and cornmeal fortified with the amino acid L-lysine.

SWEETENERS

Refined white sugar has been vastly publicized as the body's enemy and rightly so. During the low-fat craze, fat was replaced with more sugar in processed foods making them lower in fat, but higher in calories. Common sweeteners in foods include ingredients such as fructose, sucrose, and corn syrup. Just like all cheap, hard-to-digest ingredients, we consume far too many of them.

Splenda™ is a newer sweetener being promoted to diabetics. The sugar molecules of Splenda™ have been altered so your body does not react to the sugar and its effects. There have been no long term studies as to the consequence of this product on the human body. It is produced using a chemical process that introduces chlorine. To date, 3500 products use Splenda™ as an ingredient. Choose natural sweeteners versus altered ones.

▶ **Consider** that there are other delicious and healthier sweeteners that are easier for the body to digest than refined white sugar. By keeping some prepared treats, cookies and muffins made with maple syrup, handy in your freezer you can cut back on your refined sugar intake. Do not deny your craving for something sweet. Instead consider how satisfying a sensible whole organic food can be and enjoy a healthy indulgence.

You might be surprised to learn that pure maple syrup, a whole food made from the sap of a tree, is the easiest-to-digest sweetener because it digests slowly in the body. One hundred percent maple syrup is also sold as granulated maple sugar and maple cream. It does not cause a sugar rush in your blood stream, thereby allowing those that tend to be hypoglycemic to partake of several spoonfuls of maple syrup without any re-actions. For those suffering from Candida, an infection due to a yeast imbalance in the body, maple syrup does not appear to feed the yeast.

Another excellent sweetener is stevia, a natural herbal sweetener, free of calories, chemicals and the side effects associated with artificial sweeteners. It is sold in little individual "green" packets and larger bulk boxes. This sweetener tends to be very, very sweet. A little bit goes a long way.

Other natural sweeteners are rapidly absorbed into your bloodstream and can be added back into your eating lifestyle when you heal. They include malt syrups, rice and bran syrups, black-strap molasses, date sugar, beet sugar, cane syrup, cane juice, sucanat, honey and sorghum molasses.

Cranberry Spread can be made in place of store bought sugary jams. Use it as a spread on sprouted toast with soft yogurt cheese to make a tasty sandwich.

Cranberry Spread

8 cups fresh or frozen whole cranberries
2½ cups maple syrup

In a large saucepan, place cranberries and syrup. Bring to a boil and simmer one hour stirring occasionally. Pan may be partially covered to prevent splattering. Spread will thicken slightly when it cools. Remove from heat and cool. Put in glass containers with lids, leaving one inch at top. Can be frozen or will keep refrigerated for a month.

Fresh cranberries are in season and in the stores from November to January. The next best thing is whole frozen cranberries which can be found in most grocery stores year round.

WATER

Chapter 5

Introduction to Water

When creating an essential environment, the restorative properties of clean water are vital. Whether it is a glass of cool, fresh water, the soothing ripple of a trout stream, the majestic ocean waves, a clear blue lake or a nice hot bath—water is an extremely precious commodity. It is undoubtedly the most ingested substance on the planet, but at the same time, the most threatened by an almost endless list of contaminants.

Our earth contains the same amount of water since the beginning of time—albeit not the same quality. Water is gathered and stored in our seas, rivers and lakes through the hydrologic cycle of precipitation, evaporation, and run off. Forests, watersheds, wetlands and aquifers all play a role in the natural filtration process which is a precious gift of nature.

The following paragraphs will help you understand the challenges we face in cleaning our water sources. Becoming aware of these challenges will help you to take the next simple step toward the solution.

Due to population growth, pollution and excessive usage, our clean water supply has been *drastically* reduced. Today the Earth's total available fresh water supply accounts for less than 1 percent. Human intervention has disturbed the hydrologic system by leaching 2 million tons of industrial, chemical, agricultural and human waste into our daily water supply. As our earth has become more and more polluted, so has our water supply. Four million children die each year from water-related diseases. Polluted water is implicated in 80 percent of all sickness worldwide.

Rain water runs off the Earth and absorbs toxicity from pesticides and fertilizers that have been applied to yards, gardens and farm land. Heavy metals and engine fluids from cars and trucks, manure from farm animal feedlots, poisonous chemicals from mining sites and sediment from construction operations add to the polluted runoff. These contaminants end up in our drinking, fishing, bathing and swimming water.

Water is a necessity for well-being. Think of the many places and times that water touches your life—bathing, cooking, drinking, washing your dog, swimming at pools, beaches and lakes and brushing your teeth. Worldwide, industry accounts for 22 percent of total water usage; household water use is 8 percent and agricultural use is 70 percent. As reported in the 2003 U.N. Water Report, industrial water use of high-income countries can be as high as 59 percent. America is one of the highest water consumers, using more than 185 gallons per capita per day. This is almost fifteen times more than the daily requirement.

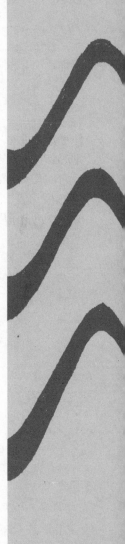

Over the last hundred years, short-sided solutions have caused the United States to underestimate and under invest in cleaning up and preserving our water supplies. It is Mr. Toad's Wild Ride out there, just like the old Disneyland attraction—turbulent and misdirected. One municipality was found to have numerous complaints from customers about the chlorine smell in their water. It turned out that the municipality's antidote for chlorine was "testing" the use of ammonia to neutralize the smell from the chlorine they had added to the water! Obviously they overlooked the warning label stating that ammonia is harmful to drink. This just encourages and confirms how important it is for you to have your water tested by a certified lab. Armed with the facts, you can then take appropriate and protective action to ensure your safety.

Distressing but true, the words pure, clean, refreshing, clear, safe and sparkling are not words that we can associate with our current water supply. We are more likely to define water as filtered, purified, distilled, bottled, flavored, sweetened and polluted. Your next step can aid in the reversal of this gloomy and overcast setting.

It is Mr. Toad's Wild Ride out there, just like the old Disneyland attraction.

Considerations for Water

It is my hope, that through education, we can develop a higher value and respect for our water and appreciate it for the miracle that it is. This chapter will introduce and explain ways to purify, conserve and protect your water. Our collective consciousness will help us to become better stewards of our water. We are worth it.

Water Related Issues

DAMS & HYDROPOWER

The United States houses over two thousand hydroelectric dams. These dams cause a disproportionate amount of damage to rivers and their surrounding habitats and wildlife while generating less than 10 percent of the nation's electricity. Dams drown vital wildlife and flood their habitats, block migratory patterns and vacillate between small trickles and forceful torrents, all of which transform a river as profoundly as clearing a forest for a shopping center.

▶ **Consider** using your voting power to prevent the development of more dams. Use your knowledge about the destruction that dams cause to our watersheds in order to educate others. Ironically, a dam is a barrier to more than just water; in fact, its name is contained in the very word that describes its consequences—*dam*age!

DESALINATION

It takes an enormous amount of energy to provide clean and safe water. One option that has been explored is the desalination of ocean water. In the past, this process of taking the salt out of sea water was cost prohibitive, but with entire regions facing water shortages, this option may now appear more practical.

Currently, salt water that has not been desalinated, called saline water, accounts for about 10 percent of all water used. It is used for thermoelectric power plant cooling, mining and industrial purposes.

▶ **Consider** that desalination technology exists and may one day be the source of your drinking water. Be aware of any new information or developments and participate in any type of legislation that may support new avenues of securing drinkable water without dire consequences.

EDUCATION

Teachers can and do play a large part in empowering their students to understand the benefits of safe, clean water. A nonprofit organization called Adopt-A-Stream is an interdisciplinary program whereby teachers and students adopt a waterway and administer chemical, physical, biological and microbiological testing to determine water quality. Teachers can select any projects, materials and activities from the Teacher's Guide that best meet their students' capabilities.

Some teachers find that enlisting a community cosponsor to aid them in their efforts is quite valuable. A local high school in my area recently received a donation from a community business to create a small ecosystem on the school's property. The students actually dug out a pond and put in indigenous plants and organisms. The appropriate wildlife was introduced and the students are now privileged observers of the natural interaction of a water system environment.

▶ **Consider** bringing this and other water awareness programs to your community. The Adopt-A-Stream program is designed to give classroom learning a real-life application, enhance students' problem-solving capabilities, and provide community recognition.

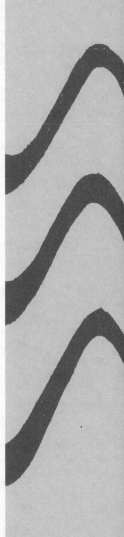

INDUSTRIAL SEWAGE

Industrial sewage is another topic that has commanded a great deal of attention and research. Let us just mention that this is a serious problem, complicated by years and years of short-sighted decisions as well as a lack of regard for our Earth. Billions of pollutants are released annually into our environments, including our waterways, from industries. No small issue.

▶ **Consider** that our watersheds, the land that protects and directs our water flow, is a valuable commodity. We all live in the *same* watershed. Therefore, sooner or later, we will all live downstream from a municipal plant or landfill. To help prevent this from becoming commonplace and acceptable, stay active and alert in your community whenever important environmental decisions are being voted on or discussed. Become a more informed watershed inhabitant and waste manager—become a better global citizen. You can take the road less traveled to create the road less toxic.

POLITICS

Be conscious of the value of our water— it is one thing we cannot clone.

Recent legislation proposes diminishing the protection for wetlands, headwaters and small streams under the Clean Water Act. Government should play more of a role in protecting the available clean water, not reducing it. Unfortunately, factory farms, and mining operations that pollute ground and surface water have powerful lobbyists in Washington that promote their agenda for profits versus safe water.

▶ **Consider** that you could become involved with the water management of your community. This will enable you to protect the policies that control your water supply. Whenever possible, vote to protect watersheds, wetlands and aquifers, all of which create the foundation for our clean water.

As change often comes from the voters, not the politicians, consider your buying habits as a vote. Buying less feed-lot meat, farm-raised fish and material goods will reduce water usage and demonstrate to the politicians what it is that you deem important.

PROTECTING YOUR WATER

We can all become better protectors of our water supply; start today. Anything you pour down the drain or onto the Earth will inevitably and eventually end up in our water supply. Over a hundred chemicals from household cleaners have been found in water treatment centers.

▶ **Consider** using free and clear household products that will reduce water contamination and your exposure to chemicals. Stand up against the development and destruction of wetlands and watershed property. Support the dedication and designation of land to conservation. Push for and demand improved pollution controls. Join water conservation organizations. Assist organizations in establishing pollution-free zones around water sources. Be conscious of the value of our water—it is one thing we cannot clone.

WATER CONTAMINANTS

The most common water contaminants are copper, lead, bacteria, methyl tertiary-butyl ether (MTBE), nitrates, perchlorate, pharmaceuticals (yes, your prescription and over-the-counter drugs), pesticides and trihalomethanes. The list of diseases linked to these contaminants are endless—birth defects, infertility, thyroid disease, cancer, endocrine disruption, miscarriages, blood disorders and more.

These contaminants leach into our drinking water from fertilizers, animal and human waste, rocket fuel, chlorination, drugs, cigarettes, industrial waste, litter, corrosive pipes and lead solder.

▶ **Consider** your actions and the actions of your associations and corporations. The contaminants in our water are mostly a result of human intervention. We need to stop the flow of contaminants into our water supply and at the same time protect ourselves from their effects. (See Water Filtration and Water Testing.)

WATER QUALITY

The Safe Drinking Water Quality Act (SDWA) was passed by Congress in 1974 to establish nationally consistent water quality standards. The Environmental Protection Agency (EPA), under the authority of the SDWA, either sets a maximum contaminant level or requires certain treatment for approximately 90 contaminants.

▶ **Consider** that even with these standards in place, drinking water and bottled water will most likely contain small amounts of some contaminants. The EPA states that people with

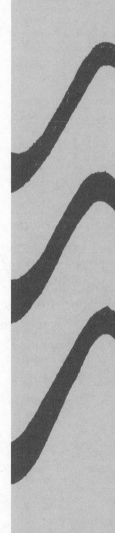

severely compromised immune systems and children may have special water needs. How about me? How about you? I have special needs too—like maintaining my own health with safe, pure water. Why should I or anyone for that matter have to compromise his or her health when quality drinking water is so important to overall wellness? The human body filters 165 quarts of water per day through the kidneys; 99 percent is reabsorbed and 1 percent or 2 quarts are eliminated. We all have a special need for fresh, pure and clean water.

Find out more about the quality of *your* municipal water treatment facility on the EPA's Office of Water website at www.epa.gov/safewater. Being better informed helps you to make better choices regarding protecting your water quality.

WATER TESTING

Contrary to what you might think, the vast majority of the nearly 100,000 water systems in the United States never or rarely ever test for the most listed water contaminants. To do so would cost most small towns more than all the fire, police and municipal services combined. As an encouragement to have your water tested, consider that pesticides have been discovered in *every* large watershed in the United States and in a hefty percentage of groundwater wells.

The human body filters 165 quarts of water per day through the kidneys; 99 percent is reabsorbed and 1 percent or 2 quarts are eliminated.

We all live in a watershed—the same one! Even at low levels, pesticides have been linked to cancer, neurological damage, and developmental problems. It is much easier to have your water tested than to find out you need to be tested for a debilitating disease—again, keep in mind the long term benefits!

▶ **Seriously consider** having your water tested by a certified lab. They can test for lead, pesticides, nitrates, nitrites, chlorine, pH, hardness, iron, hydrogen sulfide, arsenic, and other contaminants. There are do-it-yourself water tests available, but they do not test for the entire spectrum of water contaminants that could be affecting your health. Water testing laboratories are state certified, so contact your state's certification officer to obtain a list of laboratories in your state or check your local phone book for certified water testing companies. Having your water tested will allow you to determine if water filtration is needed. Depending on the number of contaminants being tested, water tests can cost from $15 to hundreds of dollars.

Contaminated water is a common source of acute and chronic illness. We can no longer assume that our water is safe.

For those using municipal water, contact your supplier for a copy of their annual drinking water quality report, sometimes called consumer confidence reports. These reports show the contaminants detected, how these contaminants compare to the EPAs drinking water standards and where their water originates. Reports are provided annually before the beginning of July. For your information and convenience, some reports are posted online. After you have read their annual report, you may need to have your water tested for specific contaminants such as lead that varies for each home and other contaminants about which you are concerned.

Water Sources

BOTTLED WATER

The fact that we need to drink bottled water brings us to the distressing truth about our water supply—*it is polluted*. Contamination of our water supply is the result of years and years of mismanagement, poor legislation and overuse. It will take as many years or more to reverse and repair these actions. You can start with one small drop at a time.

Bottled water translates into big money. Bottled water is the fastest-growing beverage category in the United States with Americans spending over $7 billion annually. Over 25 percent of bottled water is drawn from municipal sources. Although filtered to remove contaminants, it originates from the same reservoirs that supply our homes. Marketers have lulled us into believing that *all* bottled water is pure and safe when, in reality, bottled water is susceptible to many of the same contaminants found in tap water.

Many popular brands of bottled water are merely nothing more than filtered municipal or spring water. Pepsi's Aquafina and Coke's Dasani, two top-selling brands of bottled water, both come from municipal sources. As reported by the Wall Street Journal, recently, about 500,000 bottles of Dasani were recalled in England after tests revealed excessive levels of bromate, a chemical that can increase the risk of cancer. When the Coca-Cola Company introduces Dasani to the French and Italian markets, it will add minerals to the "source" water obtained from springs so it can be sold as "mineral" water rather than "purified" water that Europeans are not accustom to drinking. Interestingly, there are no minerals added to Dasani's purified water for the American market. It will not be long before someone will put a price tag on bottled water quality certification. Just like we now have certified organic food, someday we may have certified pure water.

All kinds of fancy things are being done to entice us to buy more bottled water.

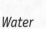

Herbs, sweeteners, flavorings and vitamins are being added to make fitness water, functional water, and nutraceutical water. Marketers are even capitalizing on pets with chicken and beef flavored bottled water. There is nothing natural about these waters. Manufacturers of these types of water are not held to the same purity standards as plain bottled water. They are not required to list a toll-free information number in order to inquire about the contents. If you want to get herbs, vitamins, minerals or sweeteners into your body, it is best to get these nutrients from whole foods rather than drink a bottle of liquid that does not disclose its exact contents.

Water coolers also fall under the heading of bottled water. Just because it is in a water cooler does not mean the water is safe and toxin free. Although the containers are made from a thicker, more industrial grade plastic that produces less off-gassing, water coolers that require these recycled plastic receptacles to be replaced are susceptible to bacteria. It is very difficult, if not impossible, to sanitize the neck of the bottle and the hands that sometimes touch the water. Water can also absorb contaminants from the air that surrounds these coolers, a fact which offers another reason to carry your own water whenever possible.

Bottled water can breed bacteria and the plastic container can give off gases, especially when exposed to high temperatures that leach toxins into the water. Even when washing and reusing a plastic water bottle it can allow potentially toxic compounds from the plastic to seep into the water. We are supposed to say "Ah" when we slug down a mouthful of water to quench our thirst, not "Ugh!"

The reason for expiration dates and regulated storage procedures for bottled water is another debated topic. Although New Jersey is the only state that requires expiration dates on bottled water, most water companies find it cheaper to stamp every bottle. Expiration dates are a notice to the consumer that the taste of the water can change over time and under certain storage conditions. However, when you start with plastic-tasting bottled water, over time and storage you are still left with plastic-tasting water.

▶ **Consider** that the best solution would be to clean up our water sources so that our tap water is safe. As part of a closed system, our water cycles continuously between the Earth's atmosphere and our soil. Therefore, protecting our environment is the best way to ensure safe and pure water. Although that sounds like an insurmountable task, the solution to minimizing your exposure to toxins in your water begins with one step at a time—your step. Congratulations, awareness is the first step and you are taking it.

When more and more of us stop buying water packaged in plastic and begin asking for water packaged in recycled glass bottles, the marketers of bottled water will change their course.

There are numerous types of bottled water available such as artesian, mineral, purified, seltzer, sparkling, spring and well. Choose water that is bottled from the source like spring, artesian or sparkling water. Spring water is retrieved from a natural spring and artesian water comes from a well that is tapped into an aquifer. Sparkling or mineral water is another good choice as it is derived from a protected underground source.

If possible, water in a recycled, reusable glass bottle is your best option. Plastic bottles are very costly for the environment and less healthy for you. Americans throw away 25,000,000 plastic beverage bottles every hour! When feasible, fill a glass bottle or a stainless steel container with pure water from your filtered tap water to take with you. It may cost a little extra effort, but the health benefit is worth it. This is not a new practice. Until the 1600's the Tiber River in Italy was drinkable—like spring water, and people took containers of it with them when traveling.

When more and more of us stop buying water packaged in plastic and begin asking for water packaged in recycled glass bottles, the marketers of bottled water will change their course.

If you are still going to grab for that plastic bottle of water, at least call the required toll-free number on the label and ask about the company's water source, purification methods, bottling, and shipping practices. It is up to the consumer to turn the tide toward water in glass containers.

And one more thing, if you are purchasing a bottle of water, unless you know the vendor, make sure the clerk or waiter hands you the bottle without unscrewing the top. This will insure your protection from a possible reused and refilled bottle of water.

CITY WATER

There are over 700 chemicals found in city drinking water. An estimated 7 million people get sick every year from drinking contaminated tap water. For more than eighty years, chlorination has been regularly used in municipal water treatment as a disinfectant. As a result, most public water in America contains by-products of chlorination that have been linked to bladder and rectal cancer. The decision to add chlorine to our water supply was based on a need to destroy disease-producing bacteria and other harmful organisms that may be present in water. Chlorine kills bacteria, but it leaves behind volatile organic chemicals (VOCs) that are extremely harmful to humans. Over the years, chlorinated water has lead to the deterioration of many water system infrastructures and the health of their citizens.

The solution to our polluted water is not an easy one by any measure, but everyone can start by increasing our protection of water and by decreasing our usage. We must find alternate ways to keep our water supply safe from bacteria, contaminants and short-sightedness.

Chlorine testing of the municipal water system by officials is a bit tricky. The tests are conducted on the dwelling farthest away from the treatment plant to insure that water does not contain bacteria or have high chlorine residual levels. Unfortunately, this practice results in the residences nearest the plant to be overdosed with chlorine so those at the end of the line receive bacteria-free water.

▶ **Consider** that the long-term goal is to clean up city water and stop harmful pollution. But in the meantime, if your tap water exposes you to toxic chemicals, then your only defense is to filter your water and carry your water with you in a glass or stainless-steel container.

As our body's largest organ, the skin absorbs chemicals six times faster topically than by ingesting them.

At the present time, find out *your* city's water quality by requesting a copy of its annual water quality report, sometimes called a right-to-know report or a consumer confidence report. This report will give you an idea of your water's quality.

Take your water to be tested at a certified lab. (See Water Testing.) The next step is to compare the results of the certified lab with the results of the city report. Believe the certified lab report. Once you know what is in the water you will know what and how to filter out contaminants.

After that, you can select a water filtration system to eliminate the particular contaminants that are present in your tap water. Just as we are advised to get second opinions from medical sources, it is a good idea to obtain at least three opinions from different water filtration companies before you make your decision.

Whole-house water systems provide safe water with the majority of them incorporating activated carbon filters which extracts chlorine from the water supply. Other household filtration methods include reverse osmosis, chlorination, ozonation, aeration and point-of-use distillation. (See Water Filtration Systems.) Always make sure to follow the manufacturer's operating and maintenance instructions.

WELL WATER

Determine the quality of your water. Have your water tested by a certified lab for harmful bacteria and chemicals, such as lead, arsenic, pathogens, trihalomethanes, halo acetic acids, radon and rocket fuel. (See Water Testing.)

Once you identify the contaminants present in your water, select and install a water filtration system to eliminate any toxins and to kill bacteria. Everyone, especially children, pregnant women and people with chronic illness need safe, clean water to thrive. If you are already using a water filtration system, make sure to conduct proper maintenance and replace expired filters. (See Water Filtration Systems.)

WETLANDS, WATERSHEDS & AQUIFERS

Wetlands, watersheds and aquifers are fundamental to our quality of life while playing a critical role in our environmental balance. Wetlands act as nature's water filters, removing impurities from runoff water that goes into rivers, lakes and our drinking water. About 275 acres of wetlands are converted each day for agriculture, property development and resource extraction. Even though these numbers are overwhelming and disheartening, do not give up the right to secure pure and clean water supplies.

▶ **Consider** voting to protect your watersheds, wetlands and aquifers. Wetlands recharge aquifers which in turn store 97 percent of the world's fresh water. Donate to agencies, organizations and conservancies that save and restore wetlands. Wetlands reduce the effects of flooding and droughts by moderating water supplies. Support your wetlands. If you are not in the financial position to donate money, always remember that you can devote something that is priceless—your time and energy!

Water Usage

BATHS AND SHOWERS

As our body's largest organ, the skin absorbs chemicals six times faster topically than by ingesting them. You certainly will not want to bathe or shower in your tap water if it is not clean and safe from toxic chemicals. The bad news is that most public water systems utilize chlorine to kill bacteria; a dangerous combination which can react with organic matter to form carcinogenic trihalomethanes (THMs). When showering, the THMs are inhaled and absorbed through your skin. They cause exposure to a higher risk of liver damage, bladder and rectal cancer.

▶ **Seriously, consider** having your water tested. Based on your findings, filter the water you use for bathing and drinking. If resources permit, a whole house filtration system is the

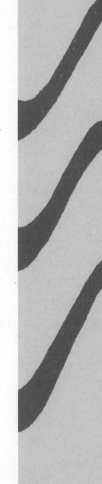

most effective. Point-of-use or absorption filtration is the next best option. Installing a filtration unit on your shower and tub can significantly reduce your exposure to unhealthy chemicals. (See Water Testing and Water Filtration.) Whenever possible, open your bathroom doors and windows to let airborne chemicals dissipate from water vapors.

The bathroom is a great place to cut water costs and resource use. As much as two to three gallons of water can run down the drain while waiting for hot water for a shower. Take a shorter shower to conserve your water usage. Invest and indulge yourself in a solar shower. Capture your warm-up shower water in a container to use later on plants or to water your compost.

On-demand hot water heaters are great for providing hot water when needed, but they use more energy to maintain. If possible, place your water heater close to your shower or install a small five- to ten-gallon hot water heater close to your bathroom. Hot water re-circulators keep hot water circulating through the pipes from the heater to the farthest fixture. The water is always hot and there is no waste waiting for it to become warm. Install a timer so circulation occurs only during shower time. Also available are gray water heat exchangers that capture the heat of the wash water and transfer it back into the water heaters. Make sure to insulate pipes to add further conservation to your water system.

Showerhead aerators pressurize tap water flow and mix with air to produce a steam that gives a satisfying yet water-saving shower. These showerheads can result in 70 percent less water usage. Choose one that has a shut-off valve so you can turn off the flow while lathering and shaving. These aerators act as flow restrictors without sacrificing the naturally invigorating shower experience. Faucet aerators are also available.

BIRD BATHS
Our little feathered friends need fresh water, too.

▶ **Consider** placing a basin of fresh, clean water in your garden or on your deck for the birds if you do not have water on your property. Refresh as needed to prevent algae or slime. Heated water receptacles are also available for those long, cold winters—not all birds fly south.

DEHYDRATION
About 75 percent of Americans are chronically dehydrated. Dehydration occurs when the body does not get enough water. Dehydration causes stress, and stress causes further de-

"Stay off the Grass for 24 Hours," *definitely screams,* *"Beware of toxicity!"*

Come on, you and I are smarter than that!

hydration. Chronic dehydration is at the root of many serious diseases. Research indicates that drinking eight to ten glasses of water daily may significantly ease back and joint pain as well as daytime fatigue.

▶ **Consider** that every function of your body is monitored and regulated by the efficient flow of water. A mere 2 percent drop in body fluids can trigger fuzzy short-term memory, among other things. Pay attention throughout the day to make sure your body is being adequately hydrated with pure water. Listen to your body as it will tell you when it needs to be hydrated. Do not over consume water either as this can deplete your body of important vitamins and minerals.

LANDSCAPES, GARDENS & YARDS

Every year enormous amounts of water are wasted from watering lawns, plants and gardens. Sprinklers drain the earth's wells and aquifers. Huge amounts of water are unnecessarily poisoned each year from synthetic fertilizers applied to yards and gardens. The fact that the lawn chemical companies place signs in the yard after they spray warning, "Stay off the Grass for 24 Hours," definitely screams, "Beware of toxicity!" Again, we have been lulled into believing that the perfect, weed-free lawn is the route to happiness. Come on, you and I are smarter than that!

▶ **Consider** protecting yourself, your children, pets and neighbors from these chemicals by not putting them on your yard or landscape. Your yard will become a safe place not only for humans but for wildlife too. What is there not to like about a few wonderful dandelions? Make some dandelion tea or pick a cute little bunch for fun; let the dandelion be the symbol that represents a chemical free lawn. You can break the paradigm that we need chemically-produced and maintained landscapes by not allowing chemically-laden runoff to pollute our community's water source.

Planting indigenous foliage, vegetation and ornamental grasses in your yard can conserve water. This is especially important in dry, arid climates where lawns take an enormous amount of water to grow and maintain. Native plants are more likely to survive and thrive on natural rainwater. You will be pleasantly surprised to see what delightful display indigenous and drought-resistant plants can create for your pleasure and those of your neighbors. Install drip irrigation for your yard and garden to conserve your water usage, using sprinklers at night rather than during the day. Use your free and clear gray water (free of chemicals and clear of dyes) on your plants that has been recycled from your bath or laundry.

LIVESTOCK

Generally you might not think that livestock would be a concern in this water chapter, but livestock production, including fish, constitutes almost 50 percent of all water usage in the U.S. It takes 2,500 gallons of water to produce one pound of meat versus 25 gallons to grow a pound of grain. Eighty-five percent of our topsoil erosion is directly associated with the raising of livestock. To add to this sad scenario, when animal wastes and fertilizers make contact with water, they become nitrites and nitrates which are known toxins.

When available, wild and free-range meat and wild fish are a better choice.

▶ **Consider** that one of your contributions to water conservation would be to eat less meat and farm-raised fish. When available, wild and free-range meat and wild fish are a better choice. To add more protein to your diet, incorporate an ancient grain called quinoa (keen-wa) into your eating lifestyle. Quinoa is a complete protein that is delicious, nutritious, easy-to-digest and quick cooking.

PERSONAL WATER CONSERVATION

Humans require about 50 quarts of water a day for drinking, bathing, cooking and other basic needs. At present, over 1 billion people lack access to clean drinking water and over 2 billion people lack adequate water sanitation. The future holds serious water shortages unless each of us considers that we are the solution and act according to our abilities.

▶ **Consider** that you could personally reduce your water usage, conserve fresh water and support your essential environment by adopting the suggestions listed below.

- *Consume less material goods.*
- *Take a shorter shower—it can save from two to seven gallons per minute.*
- *Turn off the water while you are brushing your teeth or shaving-it can save four to ten gallons per day.*
- *Run your dishwasher and washing machine only when fully loaded—it can save up to fifteen gallons per cycle.*

- Fill a gallon container with water and submerge it in your toilet tank or place a brick inside the tank—it can save a gallon for each flush.
- Fix any dripping faucets—a single drip can waste hundreds of gallons of water per week.
- Use cold water when cooking as it boils just as fast as hot water.
- Water your garden only when needed, ideally in the early morning or evening.
- Avoid watering your lawn on windy, rainy or very hot days.
- Choose to plant more shrubs and ground cover in lieu of grass as they use fewer resources, maintenance and water while providing year-round greenery.
- Buy plants that are drought-resistant. To water house plants, use "gray," warm-up, free and clear dish water or bath water.
- Place natural mulch around flowers, shrubs, vegetables and trees to reduce evaporation and to promote plant growth.
- Use soaker hoses in your garden and for shrubs to provide a slow trickle that will soak the roots and cause less evaporation.
- Install water- and energy-efficient appliances and fixtures like dishwashers, washing machines, toilets and fixtures.
- Collect rain water in a rain barrel or cistern from downspouts for use in your yard.
- If you like cold water, keep a pitcher in your refrigerator instead of running the tap until the water gets cold.
- Wash fruits and vegetables in a basin instead of under running water-it can save two to four gallons per day.
- Install aerators on your faucets that cost about $5 and reduce your water usage by approximately 25 percent.

Every little *drop* adds up to beneficial savings.

RECREATIONAL WATER USAGE

Many sports and recreational activities rely on water—boating, fishing, jet skiing, swimming, water skiing and golfing to mention a few. All of these activities and more pollute your water through the gasoline, oils and chemicals they require.

Ever wonder how clean the water is at your favorite beach? According to the National Resources Defense Council, there is no uniform national standard to protect the public from swimming in unsafe water, so beach testing and closing practices vary widely from beach to beach and state to state. Some states test for water pollution, but do not always notify the public or close beaches when testing indicates that bacteria levels in the water exceed health standards.

▶ **Consider** taking a look at your sport and determining how you can become part of the solution to water pollution and over use. For a list of tips to prevent boating pollution visit the EPA's website at www.eps.gov/otag/boat-fs/htm. To find out if a beach or lake shore is monitored and reported on regularly, visit www.nrcd.org/water/oceans or contact your state's health or environmental protection agency. The time spent learning how to prevent pollution and locating a safe beach, will improve your recreational experience whether you are on or in the water.

A cooperative effort between the United States Golf Association (USGA) and Audubon International has been developed to promote ecologically sound land management, water conservation and water quality management. For more information, visit www.usga.org/green/environment/Audubon_program.html. Suggest that the courses you patronize participate and become a balanced, natural environment that conserves and recycles water and protects your water quality.

TOILETS

A standard toilet or an older model toilet uses 5 to 7 gallons of water per flush versus the newer low-consumption models that use 1.6 gallons per flush. Some states mandate that all new toilets are required to be low consumption models. A study by the United States General Accounting Office reported low-flow toilets use 35 to 40 percent less water than the conventional or older models.

▶ **Consider** replacing your old toilet with a newer model that uses less water. Water saving toilets are sometimes called low-consumption, low-volume, water-savers, low-flush or low-flow. Since their introduction, low-consumption toilets have consistently improved in functionality. Low-water use toilets may cost more, but they can pay for themselves in a few years by reducing water usage and your water bill. You will reap the benefits of these long-term effects both economically and environmentally. Until you can replace your toilet, place a plastic bottle filled with water or a brick inside the toilet's tank to cut down on the water that is needed for flushing.

Low-flow toilets use 35 to 40 percent less water than the conventional or older models.

There are other waste removal systems available, such as composting toilets and dry toilets which may sound radical to some of you but prove to be a viable alternative where applicable. Composting or dry toilets transform human waste and toilet paper to fertilizing soil through the natural process of decomposition. It is a clean, odor-less, waterless, low-impact alternative as it does not require plumbing. Radical systems today may be the norm tomorrow—you can make it happen!

WASHING YOUR CAR

Drought, pollution and increased water usage are three good reasons not to wash your car. If you are part of the populous that desires a clean car, here is some information that will help you make better choices.

Washing a car by hand with a hose uses far more water than a conventional car wash and pollutes more ground water through the soap, grease, oil, tar and other contaminants that are rinsed off the car. A conventional car wash uses about 36 gallons of water per car versus about 100 gallons for hose washing. Some communities have fines for washing a car in the street.

▶ **Consider** washing your vehicle in a way that minimizes the impact on the environment. Wash your vehicle only when absolutely necessary. The best option, if available, is a car wash that uses recycled water. They use only 13 gallons of water which is recycled and hopefully filtered before being discharged back into our waterways. Locate a responsible car wash facility in your phone book—one that uses recycled water and filtration to protect you and your environment. You can have a clean car *and* a clean conscience!

If you have to resort to washing your car or truck by hand, use plain water and a bucket. This reduces the toxins added to the water supply and saves water. Make sure the water is discarded on the lawn, not into the street.

WASHING YOUR HANDS

According to the Center for Disease Control and Prevention, hand washing is considered the single most important act of preventing the spread of infection. Although we are trying to conserve and to protect our water supply, keep in mind that using water to wash your hands is important. Proper hand washing from children to doctors to food service personnel is an effective way to significantly reduce the transmission of disease. Think of all the surfaces your hands touch in the course of your day, from door handles to other hands; and you will quickly realize the need for proper and frequent hand washing.

Faucets are a major source of bacteria. Most medical offices have hands-free faucets to reduce the spread of disease. At one time these units were cost-prohibitive for home use, but recently some residential hands-free faucet units have appeared on the market that can be installed onto your existing faucet, reducing cross-contamination from germs and bacteria. The added benefit is that they also eliminate unnecessary and unattended water flow.

▶ **Consider** that hand washing works if done properly. As a child I was taught to quickly sing the Happy Birthday Song to make sure I spent enough time washing my hands so that they were clean. I was convinced that this was solely intended for my three brothers, but I liked singing the song. Proper hand washing includes working up lather and covering all surfaces of your hand including under the fingernails and rubbing vigorously for 10-15 seconds before rinsing.

The Center for Disease Control and Prevention states that it is critical to always wash your hands: Before eating, after using the bathroom, after changing diapers, before and after handling raw meat, poultry or fish, after touching animals, after handling money. After blowing your nose, after coughing or sneezing, before and after treating wounds or cuts, before and after touching a sick or injured person, after handling garbage, or any other occasion when there is a reasonable likelihood to pass harmful germs or viruses to others.

Appropriate hand-washing can prevent respiratory-tract infections, the number one threat to a child's health. The American military found that sniffles and coughs fell 45 percent when troops washed their hands five times a day. Hand-washing is one of the ways water helps support our whole body health.

WATER ABSORPTION

When thinking about water, remember that your body absorbs toxins six times faster through your skin than it would if you had ingested them. The skin, your largest organ, continually absorbs and excretes toxins. If you are bathing in water that is not pure or safe, it is absorbed into your system faster than if you were drinking the water.

▶ **Consider** that if you do not feel comfortable drinking your water, you probably do not want to bathe in it, wash your dishes in it or give it to your pets either.

Appropriate hand-washing can prevent respiratory-tract infections, the number one threat to a child's health.

WATER-EFFICIENT APPLIANCES

Water-efficient appliances such as dishwashers, washing machines, and toilets save money and help protect the environment. The Environmental Protection Agency (EPA) created the label Energy Star for products that meet strict energy and water-efficient criteria. Products in more than 35 categories are eligible for the Energy Star label. Although water-efficient machines may have a higher price tag, the water and energy saved makes up for the monetary difference; and the cost will eventually balance out.

▶ **Consider** the savings if just one in ten homes used Energy Star qualified appliances. It would be comparable to planting 1.7 million acres of new trees. What a wonderful image and incentive! Conserve water and reduce your water bill by using Energy Star appliances. Washing machines consume up to 20 percent of a household's annual water use. There are more than 40 models that meet the Energy Star requirements for energy and water-efficient standards.

WATER ELEMENTS & FOUNTAINS

Moving water as a decorative element can be a soothing and peaceful experience. Unfortunately, energy is usually needed to create this scenario; for some people, this is an indispensable trade off.

▶ **Consider** using distilled water in your fountain as it will stay clean longer. Never use chemicals to clean your water element. If necessary, clean with free and clear dish detergent only. If your water element is large enough, add a few aquatic plants to keep the water clean and safe for animals.

If you have a pond, most home stores sell a solar-powered fountain pump to keep water moving. They also sell earth- and animal-friendly pond purifiers. Save energy and expend some of your own physical energy by taking a walk or a hike into the woods or forest and sit near a stream and listen to nature at work.

WATER FILTRATION

Unfortunately, there are no perfect water filtration systems. However, there are systems that will significantly reduce your exposure to harmful chemicals while maintaining your health. The processes used to filter and purify water include distillation, micro-filtration, chlorination, aeration, ozonation, and absorption. Ultra-violet light kills bacteria but does

not filter water. Water filtration methods can be combined to achieve pure, safe water. The chemicals and minerals present in the water and the resources that are available to purchase a filtration system will determine the type of system you select. First, have your water tested to determine what needs to be filtered. (See Water Testing.)

Distillation involves heating water into steam so the chemicals and minerals can be precipitated out before being transformed back into water. Distilled water is the purest water with zero total dissolved solids (TDS), the measure which is used to determine if water is pure. The advantage of distillation is that the result is 100 percent pure water, while the disadvantage is that it has a high energy cost and the process can result in metal-tasting water. Also, because the process is slow and a holding tank is usually required, distillation is not the most practical or economical option for home water purification systems.

Micro-filtration or reverse osmosis results in water containing zero to five TDS which is almost pure water. It uses less energy than distillation, but involves a higher water usage. Reverse osmosis (RO) systems are designed to reduce inorganic materials from water by forcing it through a synthetic semi-permeable membrane under high pressure. RO systems vary in their ability to remove contaminants. Water pressure, water temperature, bacteria, total dissolved solids and the pH factor of the tap water affect the performance. An RO system flushes contaminates out of the water with added quantities of water which in turn, increases your water usage. Filters must be replaced regularly to avoid clogged membranes and possible contamination from bacteria.

Chlorination systems provide a chemical-feed into the water to kill bacteria and sanitize the water. When paired with a reverse osmosis system, the chlorination system provides safe water for household use while the reverse osmosis system is used for the drinking water. Unlike municipal water systems, residential chlorination processes remove the chlorine and other harmful chemicals with a recyclable carbon filter.

Ozonation is basically an active form of oxygen that oxidizes bacteria, algae, viruses and impurities in water. It has the same result as chlorine, but without the chemicals. Water passes over an electronically charged plate with enough contact time for contaminants to be filtered into a carbon medium.

The chemicals and minerals present in the water and the resources that are available to purchase a filtration system will determine the type of system you select.

Aeration is used to remove gases, such as hydrogen sulfide, methane and radon from water. Air pumps are used to oxidize water that is then run through a carbon filter to remove impurities. This process does not kill bacteria but can be combined with another system to remove the impurities.

Absorption or point-of-use filters reduce most of the worrisome organic compounds such as pesticides and benzene, chlorine, radon and lead. However, they do not remove or reduce inorganic substances. These filters come in many styles— from pitchers, to under-the-sink models, faucet-mount and shower heads. Read the packaging, as brands differ in their effectiveness and the contaminants they restrict. Never the less, if other water purification systems are not available to you absorption filters are a convenient and economical way to remove most harmful contaminants. At the very least install them at your kitchen sink and shower or bath. It is important to remember that carbon can become a breeding ground for bacteria if cartridges are not changed as recommended. Water from a well does not contain the chlorine of municipal water so it tends to breed bacteria in a carbon filter. There is a different filter for well and municipal water sources. Ask suppliers what chemicals, minerals and contaminants their filters target. Make sure to change filters as recommended.

Ceramic filters are infused with silver to inhibit the growth of bacteria. Unlike most activated carbon filters, the tiny pore size of the ceramic filter removes virtually all parasites. Some have filter attachments to effectively remove fluoride, chlorine, chemicals and lead. Again, have your water tested first to determine your water filtration needs. When purchasing a ceramic filter, choose one with stainless-steel housing.

Ultra-violet light sterilization will kill bacteria, but will not filter impurities or chemicals from water. For safety, a monitor can be installed to measure the intensity of the light to assure that it is killing the bacteria. It also notifies the user when the bulb needs to be replaced, usually about once a year. The cost of running this system 24/7 is about the same as a fluorescent light bulb. This process is ideal for water that does not need chemicals to be filtered or water that has already been filtered such as in some swimming pools.

Boiling water to purify it is often recommended for killing bacteria. While this may be true, boiling only concentrates the chemicals that may be present in the water, such as heavy metals, pesticides and fertilizer residue. Use this only in an emergency situation.

▶ **Consider** all of the filtration and purification systems and select one that best reduces your exposure to contaminants. Get opinions from three water filtration companies and weigh the pros and cons of each system based on your needs. Whatever system you select, remember to service it regularly and replace the filter as outlined by the manufacturer.

WATER HEATERS

As it does for other appliances, Energy Star does not recommend any energy-efficient water heaters. The Department of Energy was unable to give us a clear answer as to why, but told us that they most likely will revisit this issue in the future. For now, the American Council for an Energy-Efficient Economy has a list of top-rated water heaters on their website at www.aceee.org.

Tank-less water heaters are a newer alternative and can be very effective when the circumstances warrant.

▶ **Consider** other alternatives to the conventional water heaters. Tank-less water heaters are a newer alternative and can be very effective when the circumstances warrant. Tank-less water heaters use a microprocessor to electrically provide hot water only when the faucet is in use. They provide quick hot water on demand using less energy and water. (See Sources.)

Solar water heaters can be a sound environmental option but you will need to contact a solar energy system expert to see if your home and climate are feasible. (See Sources.)

WATER SOFTENERS

If you have hard water which contains a high mineral content, a water softener can protect your pipes from a build up of these minerals. The mineral build up can cause the loss of heating efficiency precipitate the need to repair and replace appliances. Water softeners have little effect on bacteria and they do not remove harmful chemicals.

Conventional water softeners, called ion exchange systems, remove the hard minerals by using resins charged with either sodium or potassium in exchange for the minerals, calcium and magnesium that make water hard. These units work but use electricity and require regular refilling with salt or potassium pellets.

Electronic, magnetic and electro-magnetic water conditioners use electromagnetic waves that pass through the pipes to polarize salt molecules in water. The debate continues about the effectiveness of this technology for softening water. Much of it depends on the strength of the magnets.

Another water softening process is polyphosphate; a chemical is added to water to stop the precipitation of new mineral build up. Unfortunately, this process does not remove existing mineral build up and the cartridges need to be replaced regularly.

▶ **Consider** using a water softener if needed, but understand that it softens water, but does not eliminate harmful chemicals or bacteria.

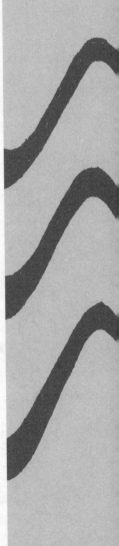

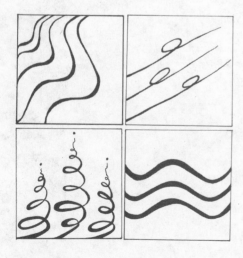

Chapter 6

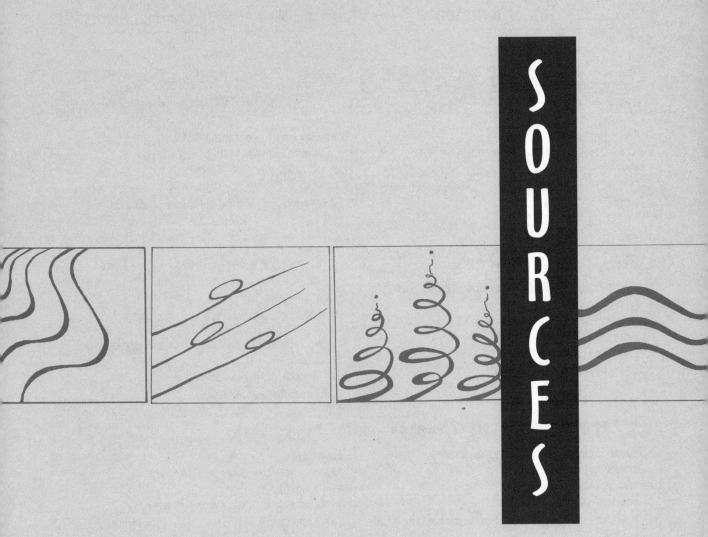

SOURCES

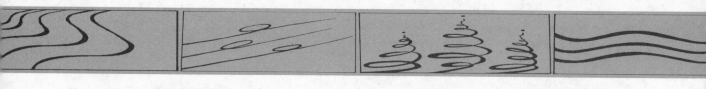

Chapter 1: You & Your Space — Earth- and human-friendly companies and products

Environmental Disorder—Chemical Sensitivity

Human Ecology Action League (HEAL)
PO Box 29629, Atlanta, GA 30359-1126
A nonprofit organization providing and encouraging healthy lifestyles that minimize potentially hazardous environmental exposure

Essential Eating

Essential Eating, a Cookbook: Discover How To Eat, Not Diet
Janie Quinn
Waverly, PA, Azure Moon Publishing, 2001
www.essentialliving.com
A wonderful guide to weight loss and restoring your health without gimmicks

Feng Shui, Ancient Art of Balance

Wind And Water: Your Personal Feng Shui Journey
Carole J. Hyder
Freedom, CA, The Crossing Press, 1998
www.crossingpress.com
Simple Feng Shui suggestions that can be done on a daily basis

Raising Corporate and Consumer Consciousness

American Environmental Outfitters, Inc.
27 Stauffer Industrial Park, Taylor, PA 18512
800 397-0292 / Fax 570 562-2885
www.aeoink.com
Screen printed and embroidered organic promotional clothing and bags

Co-op America
1612 K Street NW, Suite 600, Washington, D.C. 20006
202 872-5307 / Fax 202 331-8166
www.coopamerica.org
Building an economy for people and the planet

Developing Ecological Consciousness: Path to a Sustainable World
Christopher Uhl
Lamham, MD, Rowman & Littlefield Publishing, Inc., 2004
Professor of Biology at Pennsylvania State University, Christopher Uhl, presents the essential tools necessary for both planetary and personal transformation

Ecoworld.com
4526 Kenneth Avenue, Fair Oaks, CA 95628
916 961-6770
www.ecoworld.com / sales@ecoworld.com
An information resource on natural and clean technology

Greenhome.com
San Francisco, CA
415 282-6400
www.greenhome.com / help@greenhome.com
Online shop for green products; Green Home makes it easier to make green choices

Green Resource Center
2801 21st Avenue, Suite 110, Minneapolis, MN 55407
612 278-7100 / Fax 612 278-7101
www.greeninstitute.org / alambert@greeninstitute.org
Creating economic opportunity through sustainable community development

Natural Home Magazine
201 East Fourth Street, Loveland, CO 80537
800 340-5846
www.naturalhomemagazine.com
How to live green and healthy

The Cultural Creatives: How 50 Million People are Changing the World
Authors Paul H. Raymond, Ph.D., and
    Sherry Ruth Anderson, Ph.D.
New York, NY, Three Rivers Press, 2000.
www.randomhouse.com
"Essential reading for understanding the converging forces for profound social change in the coming decades"

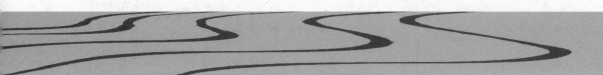

Chapter 2: Earth — Companies that support the home, office or land

Home Accessories

APPLIANCES
see ENERGY

ARTS AND CRAFTS

Budget Art Supply
11960 Mentzer Trail, Lindstrom, MN 55405
651 257-3198
www.BudgetArtMaterials.com / info@BudgetArtMaterials.com
Non toxic arts and crafts supplies

Dixon Ticonderoga Company
195 International Parkway, Heathrow, FL 32746
800 824-9430 / Fax 800 232-9396
www.dixonusa.com
Earth-friendly office supplies, pens, pencils, erasers, and Prang crayons

Near Sea Naturals
PO Box 345, Rowe, NM 87562
877 573-2913
www.nearseanaturals.com / nearsea@nearseanaturals.com
Organic, natural fabric and sewing notions

BED LINENS, BLANKETS AND TOWELS

Green Sleep
50 Colonnade Road, Ottawa, Canada ON K2E 7J6
613 727-5337 / Fax 613 727-1857
www.greensleep.com / jean@greensleep.com
Organic cotton bedding

Mother Earth Pillows
2024 Key West Drive, Suite E, Arnold, MO 63010
314 316-7075 / Fax 636 282-9517
www.motherearthpillows.com /
   info@motherearthpillows.com
Bed linens, pillows, and more

CUT FLOWERS

Organic Bouquet, Inc
242 Redwood Highway, Mill Valley, CA 94941
877 899-2468 / Fax 415 883-0754
www.organicbouquet.com
Online organic cut flower arrangements

FURNITURE

Furnature
86 Coolidge Avenue, Watertown, MA 02472
800 326-4895
www.furnature.com
Healthful upholstered furniture and mattresses

MATTRESSES & PILLOWS

Lifekind Products
800 284-4983
www.lifekind.com
Organic mattresses and bedding

Nirvana Safe Haven
3441 Golden Rain Road, Suite 3, Walnut Creek, CA 94595
800 968-9355 / 888 267-4600 / Fax 925 938-9019
www.nontoxic.com
Organic cotton, wool, latex, mattresses, futons, adjustable beds, mattress covers, pads, bedding, and pillows

Vivetique
615 847-6563
www.vivetique.com
Natural bedroom sleep systems made from organic cotton, wool and natural latex

Home Maintenance

CLEANING CLOTHS, SPONGES & PAPER TOWELS

Better Basics for the Home
Annie Berthold—Bond
New York, NY, Three Rivers Press, 1999
www.randonhouse.com
Contains 868 formulas for creating safe and healthy household products

Green & Clean
190 Highland Avenue, Athens, GA 30606
770 335-9073 / Fax 706 559-7338
www.greencleanhome.com
Sponges shine mop, tire buckets, feather dusters and scrub sponges

Nature's Way Tissue Corporation
2079-A Lawrence Drive, DePere, WI 54115
920 983-3490 / Fax 920 983-8387
www.purelycotton.com / tyess@purelycotton.com
Recycled paper products

Natural Value
14 Waterthrush Court, Sacramento, CA 95831
916 427-7242 / Fax 916 427-3784
www.natural value.com / garyk@aol.com
Waxed paper bags, sponges, cleaning clothes, scour pads and products that are safe for household cleaning available at health food stores

Seventh Generation, Inc.
212 Battery Street, Suite A, Burlington, VT 05401
802 658-3773 / Fax 802 658-1771
www.seventhgeneration.com / rfc@seventhgeneration.com
Recycled napkins, toilet paper, paper towel, tissues etc. available at health food stores

CLEANING PRODUCTS & EQUIPMENT

Bi-O-Kleen
PO Box 820689, Vancouver, WA 98682
800 477-0188 / Fax 360 576-0065
www.bi-o-kleen.com / cindy@bi-o-kleen.com
Chemical- and dye-free household cleaners and detergents available at health food stores

Cleaning Concepts, Inc.
14007 Palawan Way, # 103, Marina Del Rey, CA 90292
800 866-4742 / Fax 310 448-1047
www.cleanconcepts.com / cleanstor@msn.com
Non toxic, environmentally safe cleaning solvent

Earth Friendly Products
44 Green Bay Road, Winnetka, IL 60093
847 446-4441 / Fax 847 446-4437
www.ecos.com / rays@ecos.com
Non toxic household, bathroom, and kitchen cleaners including detergents available at health food stores

Ecover, Inc.
PO Box 911058, Commerce, CA 90091
323 720-5730 / Fax 323 720-5732
www.ecover.com / ecover@pacbell.net
All types of earth-friendly cleaners for the home available at health food stores

Green & Clean
190 Highland Avenue, Athens, GA 30606
770 335-9073 / Fax 706 559-7338
www.greencleanhome.com
Sponges, HEPA vacuum cleaners, bamboo brooms, handheld steam cleaners, non electric carpet sweeper, shine mop, tire buckets, feather dusters and scrub sponges

GAIAM Lifestyle Company
PO Box 1013, Middletown Springs, VT 05757
888 813-9559 / 802 235-1022
www.laundry-alternative.com /
    service@laundry-alternative.com
Detergent free laundry cleaning capsules, dryer sheets and chemical-free anti-static solutions available through mail order catalog

Home Trends
1450 Lyell Avenue, Rochester, NY 14606-2184
800 810-2340
www.hometrendscatalog.com
Earth and human friendly cleaners, bedding and gardening supplies

Seventh Generation, Inc.
212 Battery Street, Suite A, Burlington, VT 05401-5281
800 456-1191
www.seventhgen.com
Detergents and cleansers that are non-toxic, biodegradable and free of perfumes and dyes

Shaklee Independent Distributor
www.shaklee.net
Visit website to find a Shaklee distributor near you and to learn more about their line of healthy home and human products

Solutions Catalog
www.solutionscatalog.com
Products and solutions for a healthier earth

Qwicksilver International, Inc.
618 State Street, Bristol, TN 37620
Environmentally friendly silver, copper, brass and jewelry metal cleaning plate available at www.hammacher.com / 800 321-1484

LIGHT BULBS

Seventh Generation, Inc.
212 Battery Street, Suite A, Burlington, VT 05401
802 658-3773 / Fax 802 658-1771
www.seventhgeneration.com / rfc@seventhgeneration.com
Long Lasting natural spectrum bulbs

Westinghouse Electric Company
Philadelphia, PA
www.westinghouselightbulbs.com
Neodymium incandescent light bulbs

PACKAGING

All State Packaging
PO Box 708, Opelika, AL 36803
978 623-7268
Printing and soy inks and recycled products

Mater-Bi
Novamont, Novara, Italy
www.materbi.com / generalmanager@materbi.com
Tapioca based compostable, non static products such as diapers, sanitary napkins, cotton swabs, soap holders, cosmetic containers. Plates, cutlery, cups, straws, trays, packing systems, foamed items, pens, cartridges, rulers, and nursery pots

Planet Friendly Plastics
3216 Vanowen Street, Burbank, CA 91505
888 811-8844 / Fax 818 558-4356
www.planetfriendly.com / MareHowe@aol.com
Alternative plastic resource products

Sylvacurl
1000 Porter Brook Road, East Hardwick, VT 05836
802 472-6894 / Fax 802 472-9167
www.sylacurl.com / lovinsky@sylvacurl.com
Sylvacurl Vermont Natural Environmental Earth Friendly Packaging

RECYCLING

Acid Lead Batteries Disposal / Battery Council International
401 North Michigan Avenue, 24th Floor,
    Chicago, IL 60611-4267
312 644-3310 / Fax 312 527-6640
www.batterycouncil.org / info@batterycouncil.org
Disposal locations for acid lead batteries

Alliance of Foam Packing Recyclers
1298 Cronson Boulevard, Suite 201, Crofton, MD 21114
410 451-8340 / 410 451-8343
www.epspackaging.org / info@epspackaging.org
Locations for disposing of foam peanuts used in packaging

Cell Phones Recycling Drop Off Locations
The following companies donate proceeds from recycling to charity.

AT&T Wireless Stores
www.attwireless.com
Keep America Beautiful

The Body Shop
www.thebodyshop.com
National Coalition Against Domestic Abuse

Cingular Wireless Stores
www.cingular.com
Organizations that fight domestic violence

Nextel Stores
www.nextel.com
American Red Cross Armed Forces Emergency Services Fund

Sprint PCS Stores
www.sprintpcs.com
Easter Seals, National Organization on Disability

Staples
www.sprintpcs.com
Sierra Club

Earth 911 Recycling Centers, Water Pollution & Conservation
7301 E. Helm Street, Scottsdale, AZ 85260
480 889-2650 / Fax 480 889-2660
www.earth911.org / education@cleanup.org
Disposal information for aluminum, glass, paper, plastics, household hazardous waste, solid waste disposal, and used motor oil

EIA / Electronic Industries Alliance
2500 Wilson Boulevard, Arlington, VA 22201-3834
703 907-7500 / Fax 703 907-7501
www.eiae.org
Consumer education initiative concerning the recycling destinations of electronic devices and appliances

First Alert
780 McClure Road, Aurora, IL 60504-2495
800 323-9005
Sources for radioactive waste disposal, such as smoke detectors

GreenDisk
Sammamish, WA
800 305-DISK
www.greendisk.com / customerservice@greendisk.com
Electronic waste disposal for corporate, personal, and Technotrash, especially CD recycling

Lead Industries Association
Sparta, NJ
800 722-LEAD / 973 726-5323
Lead Media Hotline, info on how to dispose of products that contain lead

Lions Club
300 West 22nd Street, Oak Brook, IL 60523-8842
630 571-5466 / Fax 630 571-1692
domalley@lionsclub.org
Eyeglass recycling program locations

Nike Recycling Center
c/o Reuse-A-Shoe
26755 SW 95th Avenue, Wilsonville, OR 97070
www.nikereuseashoe.com
Program that collects all brands of used athletic shoes to be used in surfacing athletic courts. Website lists stores that accept donations or ship them to the above address for recycling

NEMA / National Electrical Manufacturers Association
1300 North Street, Suite 1847, Rosslyn, VA 22209
703 841-3200 / Fax 703 841-5900
www.lamprecycling.org / ric_erdheim@nema.org
Disposal of mercury lamps

RBRC / Rechargeable Battery Recycling Corporation
1000 Parkwood Circle, Suite 450, Atlanta, GA 30339
678 419-9990 / 678 419-9986
www.rbrc.org / customer@rbrc.org
Disposal of used rechargeable batteries

Recycler's World Associations Directory
PO Box 1910, Richfield Springs, NY 13439
519 767-2913
www.recycle.net
Global access to recycling

The Wireless Foundation
1250 Connecticut Avenue NW, Suite 800,
    Washington, DC 20036
202 785-0081 / Fax 202 467-5532
www.wirelessfoundation.org / foundation@ctia.org
Programs for recycling used wireless phones to help raise charity funds

SMOKE DETECTORS

BRK Brands, Inc.
Division of First Alert
3901 Liberty Street Road, Aurora, IL 60504
613 851-7330
www.firstalert.com
Alarms and smoke detectors

Materials & Components

BUILDING MATERIALS

Capital Windows and Doors
Division of M.J. Home Products
650 West Market Street, Gratz, PA 17030
717 365-3300
www.mihomeproducts.com
Energy Star approved windows and doors

Chicago Metallic Corporation
4849 South Austin Avenue, Chicago, IL 60638
800 323-7164 / 708 563-4600
www.Chicago-metallic.com
Ceiling panels and shingles

The Healthy House: How to Buy, Build, and Cure a Sick Home, 4th Edition
John Bower
Bloomington, IN, The Healthy House Institute, 2001
How houses make people sick and what to do if you live in an unhealthy home

CARPETS & FLOORING

Carousel Carpet Mill
1 Carousel Lane, Ukiah, CA 95482
707 485-0333
Natural-fiber carpeting

Dodge-Regupol, Inc.
PO Box 989, Lancaster, PA 17608-0989
800 322-1923 / 717 295-3400
www.dodge-regupol.com
Flooring made from cork and recycled rubber

Eco-Products, Inc.
3655 Frontier Avenue, Boulder, CO 80301
303 449-1876
www.ecoproducts.com
Granite tile, natural linoleum, cork, bamboo, marble and slate tiles for residential and commercial use

Eco Timber
1611 Fourth Street, San Rafael, CA 94901
415 258-8454 / Fax 415 258-8455
www.ecotimber.com / ecotimber@ecotimber.com
Chemical-free natural wool carpets, organic furniture without pesticides, foams, or formaldehydes

Forbo Flooring / Marmoleum
PO Box 667, Humboldt Industrial Park, Hazelton, PA 18201
866 MARMOLEUM / Fax 570 450-0258
www.marmoleum.com / info@themarmoleumstore.com
Earth-friendly cork flooring

Natural Cork
1710 North Leg Court, Augusta, GA 30909
706 733-6120 / Fax 706 733-8120
www.naturalcork.com / info@naturalcork.com
Natural and environmentally-safe tiles, floating floors and underlayment

CEILINGS

see BUILDING MATERIALS

ENERGY INFORMATION AND EQUIPMENT

American Wind Energy Association / AWEA
122 C Street NW, Suite 380, Washington, DC 20001
202 383-2500 / Fax 202 383-2505
www.awea.org / windmail@awea.org
Wind energy information for consumers, manufacturers, utilities, insurers, financiers, and researchers

American Council for and Energy Efficient Economy
800 363-3732
www.aceee.org
List of consumer resources for energy-efficient appliances and publications

American Solar Energy Society
2400 Central Avenue, Suite A
Boulder, CO 80301
303 443-3130 / Fax 303 443-3212
www.ases.org / ases@ases.org
Dedicated to advancing the use of solar energy for the benefit of U.S. citizens and the global environment

Center For Resource Solutions
Presidio Building 97, PO Box 29512, San Francisco, CA 94129
415 561-2100 / Fax 415 561-2105
www.resource-solutions.org /
 mlehman@resource-solutions.org
Promotes clean and efficient energy use, encourages sustainable economic growth and helps preserve the environment

Consortium for Energy Efficiency
617 589-3949
www.ceeformt.org
Information on products and appliances bearing Energy Star labels

Energy Savers
Mail Stop EE-1, Dept. Of Energy, Washington, DC 20585
202 526-9220
www.eere.energy.gov / EEREMailbox@EE.Doc.gov
Addresses the efficiency and renewable energy of buildings, industry, power, and transportation

Energy Star and Distribution Program
1200 Pennsylvania Avenue NW, Washington, DC 20460
888 782-7037
www.energystar.gov
List of energy efficient appliances and suppliers

Green-e Program
Center for Resource Solutions
PO Box 29512, Presidio Building 97, Arguello Boulevard,
 San Francisco, CA 94129
888 634-7336
www.green-e.org
Renewable electricity certification program through non-profit organization

Innovative Technology
Free Play S360 Radio
888 322-1455 / Fax 800-353-5889
www.windupradio.com
Self powered radios, chargers, flashlights, short waves, weather stations, bike lights, cell phone chargers and water purification

Sunnybrook Environmental
512 South Washington Avenue, Suite 112,
 Royal Oak, MI 48067
248 797-4173 / Fax 248 435-5289
www.sunnybrookenvironmenatal.com /
 info@sunnybrookenvironmental.com
Heaters, such as the Ceramic Radiant Stainless Steel Heater, which eliminates dust, odors, noises, fumes, and stops your HVACV from becoming duct stew

Tankless
2040-A Whitfield Park Ave
Sarasota FL 34243
800 826-5537
www.tanklessheaters.com
Tankless gas heaters

The Green Builder's Catalog
Positive Energy Conservation Products
PO Box 7568, Boulder, CO 80306
800 488-4340 / Fax 800 488-4340
www.positive-energy.com / info@positive-energy.com
Water conservation products, heat recovery ventilators, fireplace draft stoppers and other energy focus products

The Solar Living Institute
PO Box 836, 13771 S. Highway 101, Hopeland, CA 95449
707 744-2017 / Fax 707 744-1682
www.solarliving.org / sli@solarliving.org
Promotes sustainable living through inspirational, environmental alternatives

PAINT & SOLVENTS

3M
800 537-9514
www.3m.com
3Ms safest stripper available at home stores

Auro USA National Paint and Finishes
1340-G Industrial Avenue, Petaluma, CA 94952
888 302-9352 / Fax 707 769-7342
www.aurousa.com / info@aurousa.com
Organic paints for sustainable living

Bioshield
International Biochemical Industries, Inc.
800 621-2591
www.bioshield.com
Healthful paints and other household materials

Devoe Paint
www.devoe.com
No VOC Wonder Pure Paint

Dumond Chemicals
1501 Broadway, New York, NY 10036
212 869-6350
www.dumondchemicals.com
Peel Away paint stripper

Eco Design Company
1330 Rufina Circle, Santa Fe, NM 87507
800 621-2591
www.bioshieldpaint.com
Natural pigments, washes, finishes, stains, thinners, waxes and cleaners

Glidden
PO Box 130, Norwood, MA 02062
800 225-9872 / Fax 781 762-1095
www.glidden.com
Low VOC paint, Glidden 2000

HealthyHome
2435 9th Street North, Saint Petersburg, FL 33704
800 583-9523
www.HealthyHome.com
Healthy paints

Klean Strip
PO Box 1879, Memphis, TN 38101
800 235-3546 / Fax 800 621-9508
www.demandchemicals.com / klnstrp@wwbarr.com
Safer paint strippers

Safe Non Toxic Coating
888 810-4180 / Fax 805 306-1821
www.safenontoxic.com
Varnish sealer, metal polish, decoupage, primer, wood filler, odor eliminator, stain removers, finishes, stains, wax, paint stripper, brush cleaner and crackle paint

The Real Milk Paint Company
11 West Pumping Station Road, Quakertown, PA 18951
800 339-9748 / 215 538-5435
www.realmilkpaints.com / dosiever@realmilkpaints.com
Non-toxic milk paints

PLASTICS

Center for Health, Environment and Justice
www.chej.org
Information on how to identify and avoid vinyl plastics (PVC)

UPHOLSTERY & TEXTILES

see ARTS & CRAFTS; FURNITURE

Near Sea Naturals
PO Box 345, Rowe, NM 87562
877 573-2913
www.nearseanaturals.com / nearsea@nearseanaturals.com
Natural fabric and sewing notions

Office

PAPER, PENS, PENCILS & INKS

see PACKAGING

Check Gallery
PO Box 17400, Baltimore, MD 21203-7400
800 354-3540
www.checkgallery.com
Recycled checks for personal and business use

Green Drop Ink Company
2 Comm Hill, Morristown, NJ 07960
877 723-3465
www.safeartlinks.com / safeartlinks@bigfoot.com
Environmentally-friendly ink supplies and other office products

Green Earth Office Supply
59 North Santa Cruz Avenue, Los Gatos, CA 95030
408 395-3975 / Fax 408 395-3965
www.greenearthofficesupply.com /
    info@greenearthofficesupply.com
Anything and everything green for the office and home

Hemp Industries Association—HIA
PO Box 1080
Occidental, CA 95465
707 874-3648 / Fax 707 874-1104
www.HempIndustries.org / info@thehia.org
A global trade group of hemp farmers, researchers, manufacturers, and distributors offering textiles, body care, food, and paper products

Impression Holding Company, Ltd.
46 LePage Court, Toronto, ON M3J 1Z9, Canada
416 638-9895 / Fax 416 638-8167
www.recycled.com / info@recycled.com
Recycled products, such as denim pencils, and rulers, pens, frames, etc. made from recycled paper, glass, plastic, aluminum, and tires

New Leaf Paper
888 989-5323
newleafpaper.com
Leads the paper industry in the development and distribution of environmentally responsible, economically sound printing and office papers

Outdoor

COMPOSTING

Gaiam, Inc.
360 Interlocken Boulevard, Broomfield, CO 80021
877 989-6321
www.gaiam.com / merchandising@gaiam.com
Natural living products including indoor composters available through specialty stores or mail order.

MasterComposter.Com
www.mastercomposter.com
Informational website with step-by-step how-to, facts and lists of compostable materials and supplies

US Composting Council
Hauppauge, NY
631 864-2567
www.compostingcouncil.org
Composting contacts listed by state

GARDENING

see YARDS

National Gardening Association
1100 Dorset Street, South Burlington, VT 05403
802 863-5251 / Fax 802 864-6889
www.garden.org / www.kidsgardening.com
A nonprofit organization to help, educate and inform gardeners

Seeds Of Change
3250 E. 44th Street, Vernon, CA 90058
888 762-7333 / 888 762-4240
www.seedsofchange.com
Organic seeds for herbs, vegetables, flowers and trees available at health food stores

Territorial Seeds
541 942-9547
www.Territorialseeds.com
Mail order catalog offering organic regionally-appropriate plants for everyone

GOLF COURSES

United States Golf Association
Audubon International Program
www.usga.org/green/environment/Audubon_program.html
Lists participating courses

INSECT REPELLENT

see PERSONAL CARE

All Terrain
Rosemont Ventures, Inc.
PO Box 840, Sunapee, NH 03782
800 246-7328
www.allterrainco.com
Sunscreen, insect spray and latex free bandages available at most health food stores

Gardens Alive!
5100 Schenley Place, Lawrenceburg, IN 47025
513 354-1482 / 513 354-1484
www.gardensalive.com
Mail order company that is dedicated to biological control of garden pests and has a Sting-free Insect Bite Protector insect repellent

Herbal Remedies USA LLC
130 West 2nd Street, Casper, WY 82601
866 467-6444 / 307 577-6464
www.herbalremediescom / info@herbalremedies.com
Dschungel Juice Insect Repellant

Quantum Inc.
754 Washington Street, Eugene, OR 97405
800 448-1448 / Fax 541 345-9796
www.quantumhealth.com / questions@quantumhealth.com
Buzz Away Spray

INSECTS & RODENTS

Garlic Research Labs, Inc.
624 Ruberta Avenue, Glendale, CA 91201-2335
800 424-7990 / 818 247-9828
www.mosquitobarrier.com / contact@mosquitobarrier.com
Garlic deterrents for all types of outdoor pests

Orange Guard Inc.
7 Trampa Canyon Road, Carmel Valley, CA 93924
www.orangeguard.com
Home pest control that is safe to be used around food, humans and pets

Whatever Works Magazine
Earth Science Building, 74 20th Street,
    Brooklyn, NY 11232-1100
800 499-6757
www.whateverworks.com
Mail order catalog that provides solutions for earth friendly garden, home and natural pest controls

Woodstream Corporation
69 N. Locust Street, Lititz, PA
800 800-1819
www.victorpest.com
Poison-free pesticides from ants to slugs

LITTER

Adopt-A-Highway
www.adoptahighway.net

Adopt-A-Stream
www.adopt-a-stream.org

YARDS
see HOME & YARD POWER EQUIPMENT

Healthy Lawn, Healthy Environment
United States Environmental Protection Agency
www.epa.gov/oppfead1/Publications/lawncare.pdf
An informative brochure on human and earth friendly lawn care

NaturaLawn of America
1 East Church Street, Fredrick, MD 21701
800 989-5444
www.nl-amer.com
Organic-based lawn care service and products; Human powered reel lawn mower

Organic Landscape Alliance
The Wicker 777 Bay Street, PO Box 46009, Toronto, ON M5G 2P6
866 824-7685
www.organiclandscape.org
Growing the business of beautiful, healthy lawns, gardens and parks

The Environmental Factor
8-133 Taunton Road, Oshawa, ON L1G 3T3
888 820-9992 / 905 571-5047
www.environmentalfactor.com
Organic lawn and garden products, such as corn gluten and beneficial nematodes that are pesticide-free

Personal Care

BATH & BEAUTY PRODUCTS

A Consumers Dictionary of Cosmetic Ingredients
Ruth Winter, M.S.
New York, NY, Three Rivers Press, 1999
www.randomhouse.com
"Know which chemicals in today's toiletries are safe, which are potentially toxic, and which can trigger allergic reactions."

Band-Aids

All Terrain
Rosemont Ventures, Inc.
PO Box 840, Sunapee, NH 03782
800 246-7328
www.allterrainco.com
Latex free bandages for adults and children available at most health food stores

Body Sponges & Brushes

Ayate Wash Cloth
Body Crystal of California
949 443-0991
ww.bodycrystal.com
Natural fiber wash cloth

Cosmetics

Aveda Stores, Spas and Salons
866 824-1553
www.aveda.com
Visit their website to find a store near you and to learn more about their mission for a sustainable earth

Burt's Bees Inc.
PO Box 13489, Durham, NC 27709
800 849-7112 / Fax 800 429-7487
www.burtsbees.com / info@burtsbees.com
Full line cosmetics, skincare, bath, body and baby products available stores nation wide

Dr. Hauschka Skin Care, Inc.
59 North Street, Hatfield, MA 01038
800 247-9907 / Fax 413 247-0680
www.drhauschka.com / holistic-skincare@hauschka.com
Holistic skin care and decorative makeup line available at specialty stores and most health food stores

Ecco Bella
1123 Route 23 South, Wayne, NJ 07470
877 696-2220 / Fax 973 696-9666
www.eccobella.com / sales@eccobella.com
Color cosmetics containing no synthetic dyes and colors

Deodorant

Thai Crystal Deodorant Roll-On
Deodorant Stones Of America
9420 E. Double Tree Ranch Road, Scottsdale, AZ 85258
800 279-9318 / Fax 480 451-5850
www.deodorantstones.com / Robert@deodorantstones.com
Aluminum-free deodorant comes in rock, form, roll-on and non aerosol spray

Home Health
2100 Smithtown Avenue, Ronkonkoma, NY 11772
800 445-7137 / Fax 631 244-1777
www.homehealthproducts.com /
   contactus@homehealthproducts.com
Herbal magic deodorants that come in roll-on and non aerosol spray

Feminine Hygiene Products

Natracare
14901 East Hampden Avenue #190, Aurora, CO 80014
303 617-3476 / Fax 303 617-3495
www.natracare.com / nancy@natracare.com
Organic, chemical free feminine hygiene products available at health food stores

Organic Essentials
822 Badlridge Street, O'Donnell, TX 79351
800 765-6491 / 806 428-3475
www.organicessentials.com / oeinfo@pics.net
Organic cotton swabs, balls and feminine hygiene products available at health food stores

Hair Care

Aubrey Organics
4419 Manhattan Avenue, Tampa, Fl 33614
800 237-4270 / Fax 813 876-8166
www.aubrey-organics.com
Natural hair, skin, body and baby care available at specialty stores and most health food stores

Naturade Incorporated
Irvine, CA
www.aloevera80.com
Alcohol- and fragrance-free hairspray with aloe vera available at health food stores

Hair Coloring & Treatments

Aveda Stores, Spas and Salons
866 824-1553
www.aveda.com
Visit their website to find a store near you and to learn more about their mission for a sustainable earth

Herbatint
www.herbatint.com
Chemical free herbal hair color and shampoos available at health food stores

Natracolor
Herbaceutical, Inc., 902-M Enterprise Way, Napa, CA 94558
Natural hair dyes available at most health food stores

Hair Removal

Kiss My Face
PO Box 224, Gardiner, NY 12525-0224
800 262-5477 / Fax 845 255-4312
www.kissmyface.com
Nontoxic, fragrance-free shaving crème

Lotions & Sunscreens

see SKIN CARE

Nail Polish

Honey Bee Gardens, Inc.
1082 Palisades Drive, Leesport, PA 19533
610 396-9225
www.honeybeegardens.com / sales@honeybeegardens.com
Natural nail polish remover

Mad River Science
2736 Clay Road, Mckinlyville, CA 95519
707 839-4729
www.madriverscience.com / website@madriverscience.com
Chemical-free nail polish and nail polish remover

Personal Care Paper Products

see FEMININE HYGIENE PRODUCTS

Seventh Generation, Inc.
212 Battery Street, Suite A, Burlington, VT 05401-5281
800 456-1191
www.seventhgen.com
Facial and toilet tissue

Skin Care

Aubrey Organics
4419 Manhattan Avenue, Tampa, Fl 33614
800 237-4270 / Fax 813 876-8166
www.aubrey-organics.com
Natural hair, skin, body and baby care available at specialty stores and most health food stores

Dr. Hauschka Skin Care, Inc.
59 North Street, Hatfield, MA 01038
800 247-9907 / Fax 413 247-0680
www.drhauschka.com / holistic-skincare@hauschka.com
Holistic skin care and decorative makeup line available at specialty stores and most health food stores

Heritage Products
PO Box 444, Virginia Beach, VA 23458
800 862-2923 / Fax 800 329-2292
www.caycecures.com / dribler@caycecures.com
Entire line of pure body oils

Zia Natural Skincare
1337 Evans Ave San Francisco, CA 94124
800 334-7546 / Fax 415 641-2437
www.zianatural.com
Natural skin care

Soap

Burt's Bees Inc.
PO Box 13489, Durham, NC 27709
800 849-7112 / Fax 800 429-7487
www.burtsbees.com / info@burtsbees.com
Natural, hand and shower soaps

Dr. Bronner's Magic Soaps
PO Box 28, Escondido, CA 92033
760 743-2211 / Fax 760 745-6675
www.drbronner.com / customers@drbronner.com
A complete line of soap products for personal use, pet use and cleaning available at heath food stores

Toothpaste

Jason Natural Products
5500 West 83rd Street, Los Angeles, CA 90045
877 527-6601
www.jasonnaturalproducts.com
Natural toothpaste

Nature's Gate
9200 Mason Avenue, Chatsworth, CA 91311
818 882-2951 / Fax 818 407-4998
www.levlad.com / customerservice@levlad.com
Toothpastes, bath products, lotions, and several selections of deodorant available at health food stores.

CELEBRATIONS

Treecycle Recycled Paper
328 E. Main #1 / Missoula MT 59802
406 549-4572 / Fax 406-549-4573
www.treecycle.net / treecycle@blackfoot.net
Biodegradable, non-GMO wheat or corn utensils, unbleached cups, recycled paper plates and bowls; paper soup containers with paper lids; unbleached "to go" containers

Wedding Connections
PO Box 7191, San Diego, CA 91167
858 270-6155 / 858 581-5044
www.weddingconnections.com
Your complete online resource for natural, green weddings

ECOLOGICALLY CELEBRATING THE EVER AFTER

Forever Fernwood
301 Tennessee Valley Rd, Mill Valley, CA 94941
888 367-3837
www.foreverfernwood.com
An organic, eco-cemetery, offering a green space to celebrate the living as well as the dead; where people can reconnect with the cycle of life

Memorial Ecosystems
111 Main Street, Westminster, SC 29693
864-647-7798 / Fax: 864-647-0403
www.memorialecosystems.com /
   sales@memorialecosystems.com
Memorial nature park specifically designed to save and restore significant wildlands while providing economical, beautiful, environmentally responsible and mainstream alternative to existing memorial parks.

CLOTHING

A Happy Planet
334 46th Avenue, San Francisco, CA 94121
888 946-4227 / 888 424-2779 / Fax 415 221-4228
www.ahappyplanet.com / info@ahappyplanet.com
Organic fiber material and baby clothing

Athena Mills
50 West Ohio Avenue, Suite A, Richmond, CA 94804
510 231-9001 / Fax 510 231-9016
www.foxfibre.com
Lynda@athenamills.com
All natural, chemical-free clothing

Maggie's Organics
Clean Clothes, Inc.
306 Cross Street, Ypsilanti, MI 48197
800 609-8593 / Fax 734 482-4175
www.maggiesorganics.com
Safe, soft organic cotton clothing from socks to shoes to pajamas

Wearable Vegetables
5306 Canal Blvd., New Orleans, LA 70124
504 486-1117 / Fax 504 486-1103
www.maggiesorganics.com /
    maggies@maggiesorganics.com
All types of environmentally-safe clothing selections

DENTAL HYGIENE

Alternative Dentistry
PO Box 5007, Durango, CO 81301
970 259-1091
www.holisticdental.org / info@holisticdental.org
Alternative dental solutions

Ecodent Premium Oral Care
3130 Spring Street, Redwood City, CA 94063
650 364-6343 / Fax 650 365-8772
www.ecodent.com / mail@ecodent.com
Powdered tooth paste and gum care available at health food stores

Environmental Dental Association/The EDA
10160 Aviary Drive, San Diego, CA 29131
800 388-8124 / 800 510-0151
Holistic dental care and suggestions

HomeDental.com
www.homedental.com
Natural bristle toothbrushes

Internatural
Fuchs Brand
PO Box 489, Twin Lakes, WI 53181
800 905-6887
www.lotuspress.com / customerservice@internatural.com
Toothbrushes with replacement heads that are human- and earth-friendly available at health food stores

Recyline, Inc
236 Holland Street, Somerville, MA 02144
888 354-7296 / 617 776-8403
www.recycline.com / info@recyclin.com
Recyclable toothbrushes that are safe and free of chemicals

Toms of Maine
PO Box 710, Kennebunk, ME 04043
800 FOR-TOMS / Fax 207 985-5656
www.tomsofmaine.com
Toxic-free dental products available at stores nation wide

HEALTH CARE

American Academy of Allergy, Asthma, and Immunology
611 E. Wells Street, Milwaukee, WI 53202
800 822-2762 / 414 272-6071
www.aaaai.org
Physicians and information organization

Health Care Without Harm
www.noharm.org
Information about medical devices that do not contain PVC

Prescription for Nutritional Healing
Phyllis A. Balch C.M.C and James F. Balch, M.D.
New York, NY, Penguin Putnam Inc., 2000
www.penguinputnam.com
Best-selling guide to preventative medicine and holistic health

INFANTS, CHILDREN & SCHOOLS

An Encyclopedia of Natural Healing for Children
Mary Bove, N.D.
McGraw-Hill; 2nd edition, 2001
An A to Z guide for childhood diseases and their natural treatments

Baby Bunz & Co.
PO Box 113, Lyden, WA 98264
800 676-4559   www.babybunz.com
Cotton diapers

**Center for Children's Health and the Environment,
Mount Sinai School of Medicine**
Box 1043, One Gustave Levy Place, New York, NY 10029
Fax: (212) 360-6965   www.childenvironment.org
The nation's first academic research and policy center to examine the links between exposure to toxic pollutants and childhood illness

Children's Health Environmental Coalition
PO Box 1540, Princeton, NJ 08542
609 252-1915   www.checnet.org/kelly
Education and information on how to protect kids from hazardous chemicals

EcoBaby
332 Coogan Way, El Cajon, CA 92020
888 326-2229
www.ecobaby.com
Organic, natural baby items including cotton diapers, bedding, clothes and toys

Is This Your Child's World?
Doris J. Rapp, M.D.
New York, NY, Bantam Books, 1996
How You Can Fix the Schools and Homes That are Making Your
    Children Sick
Help for children who are hyperactive, asthmatic, disruptive, or suffering from chronic colds or learning problems

Seventh Generation, Inc.
212 Battery Street, Suite A, Burlington, VT 05401-5281
800 456-1191
www.seventhgen.com
Earth and baby friendly detergents, diapers and baby wipes available at health food stores

Tushies & Tender Care Diapers
Delta, CO
800 344-6379
www.tushies.com
Disposable diapers made with natural fibers and baby wipes available at health food stores

SHOES

Ecolution
PO Box 697, Santa Cruz, CA 95061
831 479-4803 / 877 817-HEMP
www.ecolution.com / debra@ecolution.com
Allergy- and toxic-free hemp shoes and clothing products

Deep E Company
322 NW 5th Avenue, Suite 209, Portland, OR 97209
503 299-6647
www.emagazine.com
Shoes that are made from organic hemp that are animal skin free, recyclable, and compostable

SUSTAINABLE INVESTING

Consumer Reports
101 Truman Avenue, Yonkers, NY 10703
www.consumerreports.org
Reference guide and latest reviews on the performance, quality and affordability of any and all products

Pet Care

Ark Naturals Products for Pets
6166 Taylor Road, #105, Naples, FL 34109
800 926-5100 / Fax 239 592-9338
www.arknaturals.com / sales@arknaturals.com
Pet food and supplements available at health food stores

Flinn Scientific, Inc.
PO Box 219, Batavia, IL 60510
800 452-1261 / Fax 866 452-1436
www.flinnscience.com / flinn@flinnscience.com
Your safer source for scientific supplies that are environmentally beneficial to fish and their aquariums including the river tank ecosystems

Integrated Pet Foods / Lick Your Chops / Advanced Nutrition
1120 Chateau Drive, West Chester, PA 19382
800 542-4677
www.integratedpet.com / ipf610@aol.com
Dog and cat food and treats that are safe and healthy available at health food stores

Pet Guard
1515 CR 315, Green Cove Springs, Orange Park, FL 32043
904 264-8500 / Fax 904 264-0802
www.petguard.com / steves@perguard.com
Full line of pet products from food to vitamins available at health food stores

The Blue Buffalo Company
444 Danbury Road, Wilton, CT 06897
800 919-2833
Natural cat and dog food found at most pet stores nationwide

Wysong Corporation
1880 N. Eastman, Midland, MI 48642
989 631-0009 / 989 632-8801
www.wysong.com / wysong@tm.net
Safe and nutritious pet foods available in health food stores

PET LITTER

Feline Pine
Nature's Earth Products Incorporate
2200 North Florida Mango Road, 2nd Floor,
    West Palm Beach, FL 33409
800 749-PINE
www.felinepine.com / talktous@naturesearth.com
Safe, affordable, biodegradable cat litter that helps the health of pets and the planet; available where pet supplies are sold

Pine Fresh
Cansorb Industries
555 Kesler Road, Cleveland, NC 27013
704 278-9603
www.pinefresh.com
Environmentally responsible company who cares about the earth and the health of cats; log on to website to find a store near you

Swheat Scoop

Pet Care Systems Incorporate
1421 Richwood Road, PO Box 1529,
   Detroit Lakes, MN 56502-1529
800 794-3287 / Fax 218 846-9612
www.swheatscoop.com

Natural wheat scooping cat litter that is non-toxic and biodegradable available where pet supplies are sold

Travel

HOTELS

Ecocities.net

Environmentally-friendly accommodations

Green Hotels Association

PO Box 420212, Houston, TX 77242
713 789-8889 / Fax 713 789-9786
www.greenhotel.com

Locations and information about green lodgings

Green Tourism Association

850 Coxwell Avenue, 2nd Floor,
   Toronto, Ontario, Canada M4C 5RI
416 392-1288 / Fax 416 392-0071
www.greentourism.ca / info@greentourism.ca

A unique, non-profit organization that is establishing an urban green tourism industry in Toronto

City Spirit Natural Pages

7282 Sir Francis Drake Blvd., PO Box 267, Laqunitas, CA 94938
800 486-4794 / Fax 800 211-6746
info@naturalpages.com

Community Resources for Sustainable Living in New York, New Jersey, Connecticut, San Francisco Bay area, and Long Island

CAR RENTALS

Budget Rent-A-Car System, Inc.

PO Box 66210, Virginia Beach, VA 23466-6210
800 527-0700
www.budget.com

Alternative fuel cars available in Los Angeles

EVRental

877 EV-RENTAL
www.evrental.com

Green rental vehicles, such as electric or hybrid cars with locations in Los Angeles, Sacramento, San Diego, San Jose, San Francisco, Ontario, Palm Springs and Burbank California

RESTAURANTS

Chez Panisse

1517 Shattuck Avenue, Berkeley, CA 94709
510 548-5049 for café reservations
510 548-5525 for restaurant reservations
www.chezpanisse.com

Celebrating over thirtieth years in operation, Executive Chef, owner and restaurateur icon, Alice Waters remains committed to good food, community, and sustainability

Josie's Restaurant

565 Third Avenue at 37th Street, New York City, NY 10016
212 490-1558
or
300 Amsterdam Avenue at 74th Street, New York City 10023
212 769-1212
www.josiesnyc.com

New healthier American Cuisine with a menu that is dairy-free using mostly organic raised items; filtered water is used for drinking, cooking and ice.

Kathy's Café
21 S. Main Street, Hughesville, PA 17737
570 584-5356
Chef, owner and Essential Eating Lifestyle Cooking School graduate, provides locally-grown, organic and sprouted grain menu items

Michaelangelo's Restaurant
894 Old State Road, Clarks Summit, PA
570 586-0755
www.michelangelosrestaurant.com
Chef, owner and Essential Eating Lifestyle Cooking School graduate provides locally-grown, organic and sprouted grain menu items along with naturally sweetened 100% cranberry juice

The Green Restaurant Association
3660 Ruffin Road, Suite E, San Diego, CA 92123
858 452-7378 / Fax 954 697-5900
www.dinegreen.com / gra@dinegreen.com
Support for sustainable restaurants, supplies safer chemicals, energy efficiency products, waste reduction, recycled products, water products and more

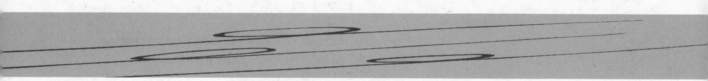

Chapter 3: Air — Companies and products that support air quality

Air Contaminants

AIR POLLUTANTS

Environmental Protection Agency
www.epa.org
Sources for state-by-state locations of hazardous waste collection website

ELECTRICAL MAGNETIC FIELDS-EMFS

Environmental Assay, Inc.
792 Green Street, Phillipsburg, NJ 08865
908 454-3965
www.emfrelief.com / eainc@emfrelief.com
Specializing in EMF, mold and indoor air quality surveys and consultations

Gardner Bender
PO Box 3241, Milwaukee, WI 53201-324
800 822-9220
Low-volt circuit alert, Item #SVD505A, detects the presence of AC voltage from 12-600v without contacting wires; battery operated

PET LITTER
see PET LITTER in Earth

SUN RAYS

Sun Solutions Clothing.com
800 895-0010 / Fax 508 540-1884
info@sunsolutions.com
Sun protective clothing

Sun Precautions
800-882-7860 / Fax 425 303-0836
www.sunprecautions.com
Sun protective clothing

Air Purification

AIR FILTRATION & PURIFICATION

Gaiam, Inc.
360 Interlocken Boulevard, Broomfield, CO 80026
303 222-3665 / Fax 303 265-9070
www.gaiam.com / ellen.feeney@gaiam.com
Filtration systems, water and air purifiers

Gonzo Corporation
800 221-0061
www.gonzocorp.com
Odor Eliminator

N.E.E.D.S. (Nutritional Ecology Environmental Delivery System)
PO Box 580, E. Syracuse, NY 13057
800 634-1380 / Fax 800 295-NEED
www.needs.com / needs@needs.com
Health and wellness mail order catalog includes a molecular absorber, water filters, personal care products, organic bedding and pet care products

Prozone
Biotech Research
7800 Whipple Avenue, Canton, OH 44767
330 494-5504
Air purifying ozone generator and ionization machine with ultraviolet light

RGF Environmental Group
3875 Fiscal Court, West Palm Beach, FL 33404
561 848-1826
www.rgf.com
Commercial and consumer education and products for air and water purification

Wein Products Inc.
115 West 25th Street, Los Angeles, California 90007
213 749-6250 / Fax 213 749-6049
www.weinproducts.com
Personal air purifiers that can be worn or used when traveling

Safe Environments
1611 Merritt Drive, Novata, CA 94949
866 896-5897 / Fax 415 382-0612
www.safeenvironments.com /
support@safeenvironments.com
Residential and commercial inspection for air quality testing services

Shaklee Corporation
4747 Willow Road, Pleasanton, CA 94588
925.924.2000 / Fax 925.924.2862
www.Shaklee.net/sunsalute
"Air Source" purification system incorporates ionization,
ozonation and ultraviolet light; large and small models available

Machines & Equipment

AUTOMOBILES & TRANSPORTATION

Biodiesel
PO Box 164898, Jefferson City, MO 65110-4898
800 841-5849 / Fax 573 635-7913
www.biodiesel.org / info@biodiesel.org
Clean burning alternative fuel produced form renewable
domestic sources

International Bicycle Fund
4887 Columbia Drive South, Seattle, WA 98108-1919
206 767-0848
www.ibike.org / engouragement/freebike.htm/ibike@ibike.org
Free bike for a day program

Lightfoot Cycles
179 Leavens Road, Darby, MT 59829
www.lightfootcycles.com / info@lightfootcycles.com
Human powered vehicles (HPV)

Xtracycle
888 537-1401
www.xtracycle.com
Customized bikes or bike kits that provide more space for cargo

HOME AND YARD POWER EQUIPMENT

American Lawn Mower Company
800 633-1501
www.reelin.com

Sunnybrook Environmental
512 S. Washington Avenue, Suite 112, Royal Oak, MI 48067
248 797-4173 / Fax 248 435-5289
www.sunnybrookenvironmental.com /
   info@sunnybrookenvironmental.com
Reel type push lawnmowers, greenhouses, composters and
rain barrels

WIRELESS PHONES

Radio Frequency Safe
2768 Cypress Drive #1. Clearwater, FL 33763
727 799-1522
www.rfsafe.com / sales@rfsafe.com
Headsets, pocket shields, wire guards and belt shields

Public Places

HOTELS
see TRAVEL

NEW CAR INTERIOR
see AIR PURIFICATION

LIMOUSINES AND CAR RENTALS
see TRAVEL

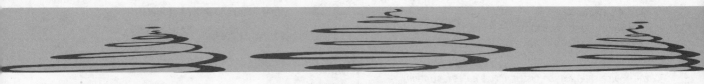

Chapter 4: Fire ⁓⁓⁓ Companies and products that support better food and drug choices

Buy, Cook & Store Chemical-Free Food

COOKWARE, UTENSILS & CUTTING BOARDS

All-Clad
424 Morganza Road, Canonsburg, PA 15317
800 255-2523 / 724 745-8300 / Fax 724 746-5035
www.allclad.com
Stainless steel cookware and bakeware with a nontoxic, titanium-oxide coating

Gold Mine Natural Food Company
San Diego, CA
800 475-3663
www.goldminenaturalfood.com
Organic and natural food, bakeware, and kitchen tools

Sur La Table
PO Box 34707, Seattle, WA 98124-1707
800 243-0852
www.sorlatable.com
Natural bakeware

Pampered Chef
800 266-5562
www.pamperedchef.com
Stoneware cookware products that are safe and nontoxic

FARMERS & THEIR MARKETS

Fulton Center for Sustainable Living
1015 Philadelphia Avenue, Chambersburg, PA 17201
717 264-4141 x3352 / Fax 717 707-1578
www.csacenter.org / info@csacenter.org
Community supported agriculture information

Organic Consumers Association
6101 Cliff Estate Road, Little Marais, MN 55614
218 +26-4164 / Fax 218 353-7652
Information on food safety, organic agriculture, and fair trade sustainability

Sustainable Agriculture Network
Beltsville, MD
301 504-6425
www.sare.org/csa/index.htm
Database of Community-Supported Agriculture (CSA) farms in US

GARDENS

See FARMERS & THEIR MARKETS

STORING FOOD

N.E.E.D.S. (Nutritional Ecology Environmental Delivery System)
PO Box 580, E. Syracuse, NY 13057
800 634-1380 / Fax 800 295-NEED
www.needs.com / needs@needs.com
Health and wellness mail order catalog offers cellophane bags for safe storage, air and water filters, personal care products, organic bedding and pet care products

Food Alterations

ADDITIVES, DIOXINS, GMOs, IRRADIATED FOODS, LABELING, PACKAGING, PESTICIDES, PRESERVATIVES

A Consumers Dictionary of Food Additives
Ruth Winter, M.S.
New York, NY, Three Rivers Press, 1999
www.randomhouse.com
"The essential guide for choosing safe and healthful food."

Beyond Pesticides
National Coalition Against the Misuse of Pesticides
701 "E" St. SE 200, Washington, DC 20003
202 543-5450
www.beyondpesticides.org
Provides the public with useful information on pesticides and alternatives to their use

Fast Food Nation: The Dark Side of the All American Meal
Eric Schlosser
New York, NY, Houghton Mifflin Company, 2001
www.houghtonmifflinbooks.com
A great read for understanding the history and future of our fast food culture

Food and Drug Administration (FDA)
www.fda.gov
List of approved additives and preservatives in food, cosmetics and medical devices

Living Downstream: An Ecologist Looks at Cancer and the Environment
Sandra Steingraber, Ph.D.
New York, NY, Perseus Publishing, 1997
Parallels the toxic chemicals in our spaces to the spread of cancer in our culture.

Silent Spring
Rachel Carson
New York, NY, Houghton Mifflin Company, 1962
An environmental classic that alerted us to the environmental and human dangers of pesticides, spurring revolutionary changes in the laws affecting our air, land and water

United States Department of Agriculture (USDA)
Office of the National Organic Program
202 720-3252
www.usda.gov / nop.webmater@usda.gov
List of approved chemicals and pesticides with standards in organic and conventional agriculture

Food Processing

ORGANIC FOOD

Brighter Day Natural Market
1102 Bull Street, Savannah, GA 31401
912 236-4703
www.brighterday.com
An educational center and organic marketplace; appointments and phone consultations available with Dr. Peter Brodhead, N.C.

Co-op America Green Pages Online
1612 K Street NW. Suite 600, Washington, DC 20003
800 58-GREEN / Fax 202 331-8166
www.greenpages.org
Locate a food co-op

Diamond Organics
PO Box 2159, Freedom, CA 95019
888 674-2642
www.diamondorganics.com / info@diamondorganics.com
Organic food by mail

Green People
420 Raymond Avenue, Santa Monica, CA 90405
310 399-9355
www.greenpeople.org
Locate food co-ops and natural, health food stores

Wild Oats Markets, Inc.
3375 Mitchell Lane, Boulder, CO 80301
800 494-WILD
www.wildoats.com / info@wildoats.com
Natural and organic food store chain

Whole Foods Market, Inc.
700 Lavaca Street, Suite 500, Austin, TX 78701
512 477-4455
www.wholefoods.com / customer.questions@wholefoods.com
World's largest retailer of natural and organic foods; currently 160 stores

SLOW FOOD

Slow Food
434 Broadway, 7th Floor, New York, NY 10013
212 965-5640 / Fax 212 226-0672
www.slowfood.com / info@slowfoodusa.org
An organization that shuns the fast food movement in favor of great tasting meals prepared from nutritious food sources

Specific Foods

BEVERAGES: BREAST MILK & BABY FORMULA

Naturally Healthy Babies and Children
Aviva Romm
Storey Books, 2000
A commonsense guide to herbal remedies, nutrition and health for children

Having Faith: An Ecologist's Journey to Motherhood
Sandra Steingraber, Ph.D.
Berkeley, CA, Berkeley Publishing Group, 2003
How to sustain and protect the ecosystem of a mother's body and the infants that inhabit them

Natural Resources Defense Council
www.nrdc.org
Information about lead paint in schools, breast milk and chemicals used in baby formula; land and water abuse; wilderness preservation

COFFEE

Green Mountain Coffee Roasters, Inc.
33 Coffee Lane, Waterbury, VT 05676-1529
800 223-6768
www.greenmountaincoffee.com
Organic and fair trade coffee available at health food stores

CHEWING GUM

see DENTAL HYGIENE

Eco-dent International, Inc.
Redwood City, CA 94063
888 326-3368
www.eco-dent.com
Sugar-free Between! Dental Gum

Peelu
PO Box 2803, Fargo, ND 58108
800 457-3358 / Fax 800 987-3358
bhansen@peelu.com
Natural chewing gum in a variety of flavors available at health food stores

Xylichew
Tundra Trading
1550 Hillhurst Avenue, Los Angeles, CA 90027
323 953-0915
www.tundratrading.com / tundratrading@aol.com
Various flavors of natural chewing gum available at health food stores

DAIRY

Horizon Organic
PO Box 17577, Boulder, CO 80308-7577
303 530-2711 / 303 652-1371
www.horizonorganic.com / barbaraf@horizonorganic.com
Organic dairy products available in stores nationwide

Organic Valley
507 W. Main Street, La Farge, WI 54639
608 625-2666 / 608 625-6206
www.organicvalley.com / eric.newman@organicvalley.com
Organic dairy products available in stores nationwide

Stonyfield Farm
Ten Burton Drive, Londonberry, NH 03053
800 776-2697
www.stonyfield.com
Organic yogurt available in stores nationwide

SPROUTED BAKING MIXES & FLOUR

Essential Eating Sprouted Baking Co.
PO 771 Waverly, PA 18471
570 586-1557 / Fax 570 586-3112
www.essentialliving.com / essliving@aol.com
Organic baking mixes made with sprouted grain flour

Essential Eating Sprouted Flour Co.
PO Box 125, Torreon, NM 87061
877 384-0337 / Fax 866 870-0776
www.creatingheaven.net/eeproducts/eesfc/orderform.html
Certified organic sprouted spelt, wheat and rye flours and sprouted spelt cereal

MEAT & POULTRY

Organic Valley
888 444-6455
www.organicvalley.com
Organic meats available in the frozen section of health food stores

QUINOA

Quinoa Corporation
PO Box 279, Gardenia, CA 90248
310 217-8125 / 310 217-8140
Quinoa grain, flour, flakes and pastas available in health food stores and mail order

SWEETENERS

Back Achers Farm
North Rome, PA
866 336-6310
backachers@epix.net
Maple syrup products

Callendar's Sugar House
Road #2 Box 174, Thompson, PA 18465-9666
570 727-2982
Maple syrup products

Loch's Maple
RR1 Box 177A, Springville, PA 18844
570 965-2679
www.lochsmaple.com / maple4u@epix.net
Maple syrup products

Food-Related Dis-Eases and Their Solutions

FERTILITY

see Earth—BREAST MILK & BABY FORMULA; INFANTS, CHILDREN & SCHOOLS

FOOD ALLERGIES

American Academy of Allergy, Asthma, and Immunology
611 E. Wells Street, Milwaukee, WI 53202
800 822-2762 / 414 272-6071
www.aaaai.org
Physicians and information organization

Chapter 5: Water ⌒ Companies and products that support water

Water Related Issues

American Rivers
1025 Vermont Avenue NW, Suite 720, Washington, DC 20005
202 347-7550 / Fax 202 347-9240
www.amrivers.org / amrivers@amrivers.org
National, nonprofit conservation organization dedicated to protecting and restoring America's rivers, and fostering a river stewardship ethic

WATER QUALITY & TESTING

NSF International
The Public Health and Safety Company
PO Box 130140
789 N. Dixboro Road, Ann Arbor, MI 48113-0140
800 673-6275 / Fax 734 769-0109
Testing and certification for home water treatment units

United States Environmental Protection Agency (EPA)
EPA's Safe Drinking Water Hotline
800 426-2171
www.epa.gov/safewater
Information and standards of your state drinking water

Water Quality Association International Headquarters & Laboratory
4151 Naperville Road, Lisle, IL 60532-1088
630 505-0160 / Fax 630 505-9637
www.wqa.org
Classifies water purification units according to the contaminants

Water Storage

BOTTLED WATER

Mountain Valley Water
Hot Springs, AK
800 643-1501
www.mountainvalleyspring.com
Fresh spring water available in glass bottles

Water Usage & Equipment

PERSONAL WATER CONSERVATION

Ecological Engineering Group
50 Beharrell Street, Concord, MA 01742-1313
978 369-9440 / Fax 978 369-2484
www.ecological-engineering.com /
   info@ecological-engineering.com
Solar Aquatics systems

RECREATIONAL WATER USAGE

BioLab
PO Box 1489, Decatur, GA 30031-1489
800 859-7946 / 404 378-1753
www.bioguard.com
Swimming pool purification

TOILETS

Envirolet USA Distribution
6391 Walmore Road, Niagara Falls, NY 14304
800 387-5126 / Fax 416 229-3124
www.envirolet.com / info@envirolet.com
Low water remote septic systems, waterless self-contained systems and waterless remote systems, including non electric, battery and electric models

WATER-EFFICIENT APPLIANCES

The Green Builder's Catalog
Positive Energy Conservation Products
PO Box 7568, Boulder, CO 80306
800 488-4340 / Fax 800 488-4340
www.positive-energy.com / info@positive-energy.com
Heat recovery ventilators, fireplace draft stoppers and other energy saving products

WATER FILTRATION

CWR, Environmental Protection Products, Inc.
100 Carney Street, Glen Cove, NY 11542
800 444-3563 / Fax 516 674-3788
www.cwrenviro.com
Doulton ceramic water filter

Healthgoods
PO Box 6463, Manchester, NH 03108-6463
888 666-7761 / Fax 603 666-0526
www.healthgoods.com / info@healthgoods.com
Electrochemical removal of chlorine, shower fixtures, water testing and drinking water filters

PUR
Air Delights
PO Box 91424, Portland, OR 97291
800 440-5556
Water filtration systems available at stores nationwide

PureAyre Odor Eliminator
2226 Eastlake Avenue #148, Seattle, WA 98102
877 PUREAYRE / Fax 888 870-4051
www.pureayre.com / info@pureayre.com
Water and air filtration systems

Sun Water Systems, Inc.
325 North Beach Street, Fort Worth, TX 76111
817 536-5250 / Fax 817 536-5286
www.aquasauna.com / charles@aquasauna.com
Water purification systems

Waterwise, Inc.
PO Box 494000, Leesburg, FL 34749
800 874-9028 / Fax 352 787-8123
www.waterwise.com / domsales@waterwise.com
Water distillers and purification systems, steam distillation, carbon filtration

WATER HEATERS

see ENERGY SOURCES

Environmental Alternative / Aqua Alternatives
2131 East Middle Drive, Freeland, WA 98249-9516
360 730-7992 / Fax 240 250-5895
www.enviroalternatives.com / petrich@whidbey.com
A large variety of energy sources including an eco fire grate and solar water heaters

Gaiam Jade Mountain
Boulder, CO
800 442-1972
www.jademountain.com
Tankless and solar water heaters

Green Depot, Inc.
6901 Bayview Drive NE, Olympia, WA 98506
360 705-2868 / Fax 360 943-6418
www.greendepotinc.com / info@greendepotinc.com
Tankless electric and gas water heaters

Low Energy Systems, Inc.
2916 South Fox Street, Englewood, CO 80110
800 873-3507 / Fax 303 781-3608
www.tanklesswaterheaters.com /
    sales@tanklesswaterheaters.com
Tankless water heaters

EPILOGUE

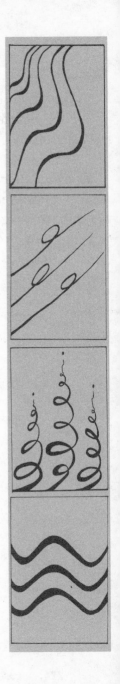

This story, called **The Green Monkey**, is another example of how their behavior is often very similar to ours.

In the 1960s a group of psychologists decided to study the social interactions among a colony of monkeys. After coming to an understanding of the social structure of the colony, the psychologists chose a monkey from the middle class of their social order. This monkey was pulled from the group, painted green and returned to the group for observation.

The monkey assumed its role in the social order, but the color of its fur made it different in the eyes of the other monkeys. It had changed and was no longer seen as part of the group. It was different. As this monkey repeatedly shared the beauty of being green, a few of the other monkeys began to accept the difference, to the point of wanting to become green themselves.

The doctors realized that humans portray the same behavior when someone in the group is different. There are human beings that are "green monkeys" and experience the same type of reactions from their fellow humans. Just like the painted monkey in the experiment, they are regarded by their friends and family as being different—they are green.

If you feel like a green monkey after reading this book, congratulations! It is a beautiful thing to realize that you are "green." What makes one person a green monkey and not another? The answer to that question is simple. At some point along the path in the jungle we all get to choose which color to become. Do we remain the color of everyone else and follow them down the worn and toxic path or do we veer off the path, become green and embrace the joy and good feelings that come from considering and making the change through better choices?

We all make choices in our life, some which affect ourselves or our immediate family and many of which affect our entire community. It is empowering to make the right choice by selecting the path to a cleaner, greener, healthier environment from which all of us can benefit.

And as our friend Kermit the Frog reminds us—

*But green's the color of spring
And green can be cool and friendly-like
And green can be big like an ocean, or important
Like a mountain, or tall like a tree.*

*When green is all there is to be
It could make you wonder why, but why wonder why
Wonder, I am green and it'll do fine, it's beautiful
And I think it's what I want to be.*

If you feel like a green monkey after reading this book, congratulations! It is a beautiful thing to realize that you are "green."

May *our* jungle be ever filled with colonies of "green monkeys" choosing to live in essential environments.

WITH LOVE

It is with much love that I extend my gratitude, respect, admiration and thanks to those that pushed, pulled and cheered me on through this creative process. Creative works are always conceived through the grace of our universe, my greatest inspiration and teacher. Many special people have assisted me in this creation and I consider them part of that grace. I am deeply blessed. For without their love and enthusiasm, this book would not be the book it is today.

To my essential cheerleader, best friend and husband Tony for sharing this path with me. To my children, their spouses and to my grandchildren; Jenifer, Wilson, Quinn, Moriah, Jeff, Matthew, Queen, Erin, Eddie and Baby Roo for enriching my life beyond belief. To my fellow path whackers and best buddies Valerie Kiser and Georgia Anderson, for their dedication and open-ended job descriptions.

Much love and thanks to the very best spiritual cheerleaders, Monsignor Joseph G. Quinn and Matthew Kelly. Cheers to the most wonderful and handsome Joseph Burinsky for helping me to have a deeper connection to our earth.

To my wonderful word experts Lee Ann Cavanaugh and Pattie Franks-Evanish, for without them I surely would have put the commas in the wrong place. To Kathryn LeSoine for her photographs that truly make our world a more beautiful place. To my book design and production team, Dick Stipe, Tracy Pitz, Lisa Erb, Tony Acquaviva, Barry Friedland, Mindy Boston and especially Cindy Szili, who so gets "it." To Jean Rosenkrans for her unending knowledge. To my savvy literary agent, that I hope to have one day!

A special thanks to all of the Essential Eaters who are also widening the essential environments' path. It is the feedback on your improved health that makes our work worth-

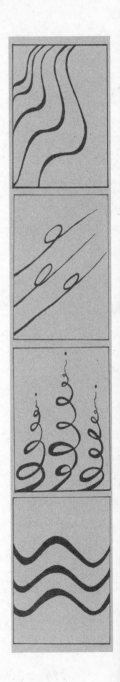

while. To Michael and Bob Suchy and Bob Lajoie for introducing essential eating to the restaurant scene. To Kathy Bender and her team at Kathy's Café for striving to provide real food that is locally grown. To Joe Cognetti and his team at Caravia's for supporting our Essential Eaters with quality organics.

To all of the specialists who gave of your precious time and technical talents—Dr. Margaret Mariotti, Dr. Gerald Reisinger, Dr. Martin Karpeh, Leon Schwackhamer, Robert Vanness, Mark Pappalardo, Rick Rippon, and Dr. Laurie Mintz. To Len Kachinski and Kathleen Calpin for their contributions that were deeply appreciated.

With much love and appreciation to my family and ancestors for being my foundation. To Bob and Susie for doing a great "Mom and Dad" trip. To Beth and Nancy, the very best friends a girl could ever have. To my three brothers, Dan, Charlie and Andy, who just like when we were growing up, did not do a thing for this book, but I love them anyway! To my bonus sisters, Rosie, Susie, Maggie, Melissa, Julie, Sheila, Rebecca, Judy, Eileen, and Brandice, all my love and respect for being such awesome women. To my over 50 (who can keep track?!) nieces and nephews who remind me daily of the miracle and beauty in the cycle of life.

I am deeply grateful to these special people for their contributions to *Essential Environments* and its concept of sustainable living in harmony with Mother Earth.

And finally, I give thanks to those that I have yet to cross paths with that continue to diligently work toward a better environment. You are immensely appreciated and I am so very proud of you.

With love, thanks, thanks, and more thanks.

Index

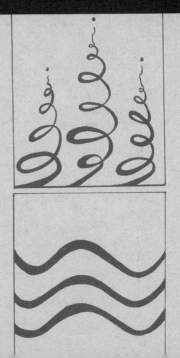

Mosquitoes, 39, 57
Mothballs, 69
MTBEs, 173
Mucus Reaction test, 141
Multiple Chemical Sensitivity (MCS)
        disorder, 7, 94
Murphy, Todd, 147

N

Nail polish, 65, 207
NASA (National Aeronautics and Space
        Administration), 99
National Air Duct Cleaners Association,
        103
National Gardening Association, 54
National Organic Program (USDA), 61,
        128–129
National Organic Standards, 135
National Resources Defense Council,
        107, 184
National Safety Council, 37
National School Lunch Program, 74
National Soft Drink Association, 150
Natural fibers, 49, 68–69
Natural Home magazine, 74
Natural Resources Defense Council, 51,
        148
Nature, as healing force, 2, 9–10
N.E.E.D.S., 122
Negative ions, 99–100, 110–111
Neodymium light bulbs, 35
Newspapers, 37, 52
Newton John, Olivia, 75
Ni-Cad (nickel-cadmium) batteries,
        24–25
NiMH (nickel metal hydride)
        battery, 25
Noise pollution, 96–97
Non-stick cookware, 119

O

Obesity, 142–143
    chemicals and, 4
    fast food and, 11
    in pets, 80
    as public health issue, 140
    school children and, 8
Office, 49–53, 203
Omega-3 fatty acids, 153
Organic food, 135–136
    certified organic label, 22
    children and, 75
    companies and products, 217–218
    consumer demand and, 10–11
    eggs, 152–153
    gardening and, 55–57
    GMOs and, 127
    as a green tourist, 82
    kosher label, 134
    meaning of, 60–61
    restaurants and, 84
Organic Style magazine, 84
Outdoors, 54–60, 203–205
Oven Fried Chicken (recipe), 133–134
Ovens, 30–31
Over-the-counter (OTC) drugs, 143
Ozonation, 41, 188
Ozone generation, 100–101

P

Packaging
    companies and products, 198, 217
    food, 129–130
    landfills and, 36
    PVC in, 47
    recycling, 37
    shredded material for, 33
Paints, 45–47, 88–89, 202–203

Pans, cleaning, 27–28
Paper products, 25, 51–52, 68
    companies and products, 196–197,
        203
    personal care, 65
PCBs (Polychlorinated Biphenyls), 48,
        147–148, 153
Pens/pencils, 51–52, 203
Penta BDE, 42
Perchlorethylene, 42
Percoethylene, 71
Perfumes. *See* Fragrances
Personal care
    bath and beauty products, 60–67
    celebrations, 67–68
    clothing, 68–69
    companies and products, 205–211
    dental hygiene, 69–71
    dry cleaning, 71
    eyewear, 71–72
    gift giving, 72
    health care, 73
    infants, children, and schools,
        74–75
    labeling, 75–76
    plants, 76–77
    shoes, 77
    sustainable investing, 77–78
    tanning and, 78–79
Personal Responsibility in Food
        Consumption Act, 132
Pesticides
    air fresheners and, 88
    companies and products, 217
    cotton and, 63
    DDT as, 126
    food alterations and, 130–131
    golf courses and, 56
    hospitals and, 73
    imported foods and, 136
    organic products and, 69

Pesticides *(continued)*
  in sponges, 25
  toxicity of, 58
  water and, 54, 153
Pet care, 79–81, 97, 211–212
Phenylethylamine, 137
Pheromone, 58
Photobiologic spectra, 35
Photosensitivity, 79
Photosynthesis, 99
Pillows, 22–23, 196
Plants, 76–77
  air purification and, 104
  clean air and, 99
  water for, 180
Plastics, 47–48, 69, 203
Point-of-use filters, 180, 189
Pollution/pollutants
  air, 87, 89–90, 107–108, 213
  chemical, 42
  cruise ships and, 82
  houses and, 17
  industrial, 95
  light as, 34–35
  noise, 96–97
  office machines and, 50
  pesticides and, 55
  tires and, 39
  of water, 169
  See also Contaminants
Polyvinyl alcohol (PVA), 22
Polyvinyl chloride (PVC). *See* PVC
Popcorn, 161–162
Posture, 143
Potatoes, 162–163
Potpourri, 97
Poultry, 161, 219
Powdered milk, 69
Power plants, 95
Pregnant women
  aerosol sprays and, 88
  litter boxes and, 81

MSG and, 123
pet products and, 80
risks to avoid, 148
Prescription drugs, 144
Preservatives, 131, 217
Preston, Kelly, 75
Processed food, 136
  airline food, 131–132
  chemicals and, 8
  companies and products, 217–218
  farm subsidies and, 117
  fast food, 132–134
  preservatives and, 131, 217
Public places, 53, 109–112
PVC (polyvinyl chloride)
  building materials and, 40
  chlorine and, 51
  clothing and, 68
  hospitals and, 73
  pets and, 80–81
  phase out of, 69
  toxicity of, 47–48

Q

Quinoa, 163–164, 219

R

Radioactive material, 35, 37–38, 89
Radio frequency (RF) radiation, 109,
  127–128, 217
Radon, 89
Rapp, Doris. J., 75
Recipes
  ALT sandwich, 132
  Banana Bread, 158
  Carob Fudge Nut Balls, 138
  Cranberry Juice, 151
  Cranberry Spread, 166

  Edamame, 118–119
  Herb Baked Fish, 154
  Oven Fried Chicken, 133–134
  Vegetable Mashed Potatoes, 163
  Vegetable Quinoa Pilaf, 164
  Wheat-free Tortilla Soup, 156
  Wheat-free Waffles, 159–160
Recycling, 36–38
  carpets, 41
  companies and products, 198–200
  green office and, 50
  as a green tourist, 81
  hotels and, 82
  junk mail, 33
  paints, 46
  paper, 51
  tires, 39
Reflexology, 11
Rental cars, 83, 112, 212
Restaurants, 83–84, 109–110, 212–213
Reuse-a-Shoe program (Nike), 37–38
Reverse osmosis (RO), 188
RF (radio frequency) radiation, 109,
  127–128, 217
Rodents, 57–58, 204–205
Romm, Aviva, 148

S

Saccharin, 67
Safe Drinking Water Act (SDWA), 173
Salt
  cleaning pots, 28
  cleaning silver, 30
  in deodorant, 62
  pet odors and, 27
Schools, 74–75
  chemicals and, 8
  companies and products, 210
  soft drinks and, 150
Seasonal affected disorder (SAD), 34

Vinegar, 26–29, 58, 63
Volatile organic chemicals (VOCs), 45,
    48–49, 177

W

Waste management
  hazardous waste disposal, 90
  hospitals and, 73
  hotels and, 83
  paper industry and, 51
  radioactive waste and, 37
  toxic waste disposal, 33, 36
Water, 169–170, 179–187
  boiling to purify, 189–190
  companies and products, 220–222
  conservation of, 82–83
  contamination of, 153
  EPA standards, 19
  filtration of, 70, 180, 187–190, 221
  hydro power, 43, 170–171
  industrial sewage and, 172
  paper industry and, 51
  personal water conservation,
    182–183, 221
  pesticides and, 54
  protecting, 172–173
  quality of, 173–174, 220
  testing, 174–175, 180, 220
Water heaters, 190, 222
Waters, Alice, 55–56
Water softeners, 190–191
Wetlands, 172, 179
Wheat-free Tortilla Soup (recipe), 156
Wheat-free Waffles (recipe), 159–160
Wheat products, 158–160
Wind energy, 43

Windows, 31, 49
Winter, Ruth, 61
Wireless phones, 37, 91–92, 109, 215
World Health Organization, 111
Wrapping paper, 67–68

Y

Yards, 59–60
  companies and products, 205
  power equipment for, 107–108, 215
  water usage and, 181–182

Z

Zero emission vehicles (ZEVs), 106

QUICK ORDER FORM

—◁◁◁▷▷▷—

To purchase additional copies of Essential Environments:

🖥 **INTERNET ORDERS:**   www.essentialliving.com. Click on Products.

🖷 **FAX ORDERS:**   Toll free (888) 267-0605. Fill out and fax this form.

☏ **TELEPHONE ORDERS:**   Call toll free (877) 771-1216.

🖹 **POSTAL ORDERS:**   Azure Moon Publishing, P.O. Box 771-10, Waverly, PA 18471, USA.
Telephone: (570) 586-1557. Please fill out and send this form.

NAME: _____

ADDRESS: _____

CITY, STATE, ZIP: _____

TELEPHONE: _____

E-MAIL ADDRESS: _____

TITLE	QUANTITY	PRICE
ESSENTIAL ENVIRONMENTS	_____ × $24.95 US/$34.95 CAN	
PA SALES TAX: Please add 6% for books shipped to Pennsylvania addresses (1.80 per book).		
U.S. SHIPPING AND HANDLING: $5.00 for the first book and $3 for each additional book.		
TOTAL		

PAYMENT IN U.S. FUNDS: ☐ Cheque enclosed, payable to *Azure Moon Publishing*
☐ VISA   ☐ MasterCard

CARD NUMBER: _____

NAME ON CARD: _____   EXP. DATE: _____ / _____

Thank you for your order.